WORKING WITH
DIFFICULT PATIENTS

WORKING WITH DIFFICULT PATIENTS

From Neurosis to Psychosis

Franco De Masi

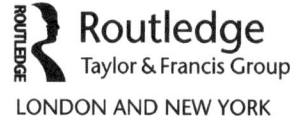

Routledge
Taylor & Francis Group

LONDON AND NEW YORK

First published in Italian in 2012 as: *Lavorare con i pazienti difficili*
by Bollati Boringhieri, Turin

First published 2012 by Karnac Books Ltd.

Published 2018 by Routledge
2 Park Square, Milton Park, Abingdon, Oxon OX14 4RN
711 Third Avenue, New York, NY 10017, USA

Routledge is an imprint of the Taylor & Francis Group, an informa business

Copyright © 2012 Bollati Boringhieri editore, Torino.

The right of Franco De Masi to be identified as the author of this work has
been asserted in accordance with §§ 77 and 78 of the Copyright Design and
Patents Act 1988.

Translated by Harriet Graham and others
Translator's note: any quotations not taken from a published English edition
have been translated from Italian, and, unless referring to a specific, named
person, the masculine form has been used throughout for both "analyst" and
"patient".

Note: Chapters Six, Seven, Nine, and Thirteen were originally translated by
Philip Slotkin. Chapter Ten was originally translated by Giovanna Iannaco
and published in *The International Journal of Psychoanalysis*. All previously
translated material has been integrated and edited by Harriet Graham.

British Library Cataloguing in Publication Data

A C.I.P. for this book is available from the British Library

ISBN 9781782200437 (pbk)

Edited, designed and produced by The Studio Publishing Services Ltd
www.publishingservicesuk.co.uk
e-mail: studio@publishingservicesuk.co.uk

CONTENTS

For Paula, who knows why.

ABOUT THE AUTHOR

Franco De Masi is a training and supervising analyst of the Italian Psychoanalytical Society and former President of Centro Milanese di Psicoanalisi and Secretary of the Training Milanese Institute. He is a medical doctor and a psychiatrist who worked for twenty years in psychiatric hospitals. Now he lives and works as a full-time psychoanalyst in Milan. Currently, his main interests are focused on the theoretical and technical psychoanalytical issues related to severely ill patients. He has published several papers in *The International Journal of Psychoanalysis* and in the *Rivista Italiana di Psicoanalisi* and in other International Reviews. He is author and editor of numerous books: *The Sadomasochistic Perversion: the Object and the Theories; Making Death Thinkable: a Psychoanalytic Contribution to the Problem of the Transience of Life; Vulnerability to Psychosis: A Psychoanalytic Study of the Nature and Therapy of the Psychotic State,* and *The Enigma of the Suicide Bomber: A Psychoanalytic Essay.*

Introduction

One of the many stories in *The Mahabharata*, the legendary Indian epic, tells of Drona, a prince fallen from grace who is taken on as preceptor to the royal family. One of his tasks is to teach the king's three sons archery. So, he sets up a lifelike bird half-hidden among the branches of a tree in the park. He gives the eldest prince a bow and arrow and then asks him what he sees. The boy answers, "I see the bird in the tree. I see the leaves on the tree. I see you, my master, and I see my brothers." Drona says, "Put aside your bow and stand apart," and then asks the second brother but obtains the same answer, and so—by now very discouraged—asks the third. This time the boy replies, "I see only the head of the bird, nothing else"; he nocks his arrow, draws his bow, and lets the arrow fly—straight to its mark, the head of the bird.

With this tale, I would like to introduce an important concept of this book: which patient are we addressing when we work with our analysand?

In our consulting rooms, we resemble the brothers in the story; we see many things (the tree, its leaves, the brothers, and so on) but we must choose only one of the many elements present, the one that seems to us *specifically* pertinent to that particular configuration–relationship–patient story.

When we work with a difficult patient, we must consider him not just as an individual with his particular history and suffering, but also as a bearer of a specific psychopathological configuration that would nullify any therapy if it were not identified and treated.

The word "psychopathology"—used to characterise the patient's conditions of suffering—is often felt to be discriminating and objectivising and so is rarely adopted in psychoanalytic communication. In my view, however, the psychopathology is the fundamental component permeating and structuring the analytic process, conditioning the transference, and marking moments of impasse and transformation. In other words, a constant dialectic tension exists between the psychopathology and the bag of tools that we have at our disposal for understanding and fostering change.

One of the cardinal points of this book is that the psychopathology, no matter its entity or on what level it is located, should be considered the perturbing and enriching element in our daily therapeutic work. Taking the time to study it once again and paying particular attention to the elements that define it can only stimulate the creation of tools capable of treating the most difficult cases.

In fact, the analyst is constantly in the position of having to increase his fields of knowledge; this holds good as much for the individual analyst as for the group as a whole. It makes psychoanalytic practice more remunerative than other disciplines, such as, for example, psychiatry, where research is distinct from clinical activity. In the analytic field, the two spheres are present in the same moment. As the patient changes during analysis, so, too, the analyst's clinical view and his emotional receptiveness constantly broaden.

The book is divided into two parts.

The first part discusses the parameters that define the scope of our work with difficult patients. I have attempted to trace out a series of connections that give rise to the intimate relationship between environment and individual in the construction of emotional suffering, emphasising both the undisputed pathogenic action of environmental stimuli and the active participation of whoever is obliged to suffer the negative situation. In fact, the way in which one tries to escape suffering is what often seriously jeopardises growth.

The first chapters illustrate the importance of trauma as the producer of pathology. My aim is to point out the intrinsic link between some forms of mental suffering and the distorted responses that the patient has received from his original environment. For this reason, I explore the concept of the *emotional trauma* in particular, since this trauma, which occurs in the primary relationship, often impels the child into relational withdrawal and to constructing pathological structures that will accompany him for the rest of his life.

Identifying the *pathological constructions* is, in my view, another important topic. In traditional analytic theory, the defences, activated to protect the individual against anxiety, lessen his vitality; however, on tackling the more complex disorders in analysis, we realise that this concept is not sufficiently adequate for grasping the self-destructive potential present in serious pathologies.

In the second part of the book, I examine a number of single "difficult" pathologies (particularly sexual disorders, including paedophilia, borderline states, and delusional structures) with a view to illustrating the relationship between the patient's childhood past and possible traumatic situations. My aim is to focus attention on the elements at work in the different psychopathological conditions and to find the key for eventually transforming them.

I have ordered the various chapters according to a scale of increasing treatment difficulty, which is proportional to the potential pathogenicity of the underlying psychopathological structure. Consequently, the borderline state and the psychotic state are located at either end of an axis of progressive complexity and difficulty towards change.

I have endeavoured to set out a panorama of the main psychopathological entities as I have encountered them, and as I still encounter them, in my clinical activity, presenting the material according to a criterion that highlights the differences between the individual case histories. A number of chapters in the second part of the book attempt to clarify the various psychic processes that underlie some frequently encountered psychopathologies. The analyst is, in fact, able to find an adequate mental setting for the clinical condition only when he has a clear idea of the nature of the specific psychopathological process and of the structure dominating the patient. For example, some interpretative styles are perfectly satisfactory in one case but ineffective, if not counterproductive, when the level of the psychopathology alters.

I hope these words will be useful for those who are interested in the development of psychoanalysis and its curative powers and, in particular, for colleagues who work with difficult patients and who aspire to attain ever more finely honed therapeutic skills.

As will be seen on reading this book, I consider the contribution that comes from knowledge of past psychoanalytic theories to be extremely important, but I believe that we still have to find satisfactory responses for our work with difficult patients.

After considerable progress made in the post-war period, psychoanalysis today would seem to have paused somewhat in its development. One of the possible reasons for this might be that analysts have recently focused their attention chiefly on comparing and integrating the various models that, for geographic and cultural reasons, have developed in diverse ways over the last decades. These efforts might well have shifted attention and energy away from true clinical research.

At this point, I would like to recall the radical point of view put forward by Mark Solms (2006), a colleague active in the attempt to integrate psychoanalysis and neuroscience. Solms postulates that psychoanalysis today has lost sight of the general picture and has become preoccupied only with itself, instead of with the mind in general; in so doing, it has lost its object and entered into a sort of self-centred relationship, rather like a narcissistic patient. His convictions, though, are perhaps somewhat limited, since they do not take into account all the recent contributions that have attempted to examine in greater depth the way in which communication occurs between the mind of the analysand and that of the analyst, what the latter's unconscious processes are that help him arrive at formulating an interpretation, and what the contribution of both is in constructing the analytic process. But that is not all: in the last two decades the mother--child relationship that will go on to structure or distort the personality of the newborn has been studied systematically and in great detail (especially through attachment theory and infant research). Particular attention and value has also been given to the carer's response in creating personal emotional significance.

However, it is also true that contemporary psychoanalysis has loosened its ties with clinical practice. Suffice to think of the increasingly frequent contributions in which the clinical material is proportionately much reduced; furthermore, when exemplifying a case history, the discussion is often limited to an isolated sequence without any further information about the patient's history or level of gravity of the disorder.

Solms envisages a possible future for psychoanalysis in a close alliance with neuroscience, but, although fascinating, this solution seems, in my opinion, difficult to put into practice since the two disciplines are different in nature and epistemologically incompatible. They can certainly advance in parallel and confront each other, but, if psychoanalysis wants to remain faithful to itself, it cannot lose its specific nature and its own method of investigation.

The unconscious functions of the mind are an epistemological object and, as such, are not specific to psychoanalysis; nevertheless, they constitute its privileged and specific field because they correspond to, and identify with, its instrument and its study object. While the function that allows comprehension of thought and emotion is unconscious, psychoanalysis tries to know the inner, traumatic, and iatrogenic reasons for its malfunctioning.

In my opinion, deeper investigation into the field of the more complex psychopathologies might represent a possible development direction for our discipline, since they provide opportunities for exploring unusual dimensions of the mind and intimate connections between emotional development and environment. In other words, readers of this book will notice that I have attributed great importance to the *patient's internal world and to his psychic structure*. Indeed, I believe that being emotionally close to the patient in the analytic encounter is a necessary and unavoidable prerequisite that fosters successful therapy but does not exhaust the therapeutic task.

Several chapters deal specifically with the psychic structures that act on the patient's internal world: psychopathological constructions, the normal and pathological superego, psychic withdrawal, and the psychotic part of the personality, to mention only a few of the relevant topics.

On the subject of difficult patients, we must not forget that the analytic technique was conceived for treating averagely neurotic patients. For this reason, we are led to apply the same method to all patients, seeking to obtain the maximum from a few elements that we hold to be the most significant. However, in the face of the huge differences we observe in case histories, we must admit that analytic technique should, instead, be conceived as a made-to-measure suit of clothes.

Proposals for adopting a specific technique for each patient have already been advanced by many authors (Thomä & Kächele, 1985), but, as Jiménez (2006) points out, have not found much success owing to a prevailing idea for homogeneity that sees the unity of the psyche emerging from a global organising principle that is the same for all components, since the mind is something that evolves as a whole.

Bleichmar (2004), too, proposes adopting a modular conception of psychoanalysis and suggests a technique with flexible therapeutic interventions that takes into account the sub-type of the psychopathological picture, the personality structure, and the stage reached by the patient in his life. In fact, we have to admit that patients do exist who are unresponsive not so much to psychoanalysis as to certain analysts who want to use a type of listening in their analysis that does not allow for the patient's specific psychopathological state. I am referring to patients who do not have an unconscious system capable of symbolising and of representing their emotional states; this is why they do not make associations when they dream and why the dream sequence remains concrete and meaningless.

Another important issue, which is generally never mentioned, concerns the limits, or extent, to which patients can be treated.

It must be said that with present-day knowledge it is easier to tackle the great sphere of the neuroses, whose basic mechanisms and paths of development we are familiar with, rather than other forms of mental suffering. The neurotic patient uses his dynamic unconscious and, thus, permits an analytic approach whose keystone remains the interpretation of dreams, defences, and splits.

I believe that further exploration of the realm of the structures that prevent the unconscious from being used normally would allow us to get closer to the unsolved mystery of more complex pathologies and to see the functioning of the mind with new eyes, detecting links, processes, and psychic realities that are not codified by traditional metapsychology.

This book aims to widen the research and the application of analytic therapy to those patients who, in highlighting our limits, can only take the name of *difficult patients*.

There is a vast difference between those patients who have had satis-factory early experiences which can be discovered in the transference, and those whose very early experiences have been so deficient or distorted that the analyst has to be the first in the patient's life to supply certain environmental essentials. (Winnicott, 1975, p. 197)

PART I

PART I

CHAPTER ONE

What do we mean by difficult patients?

"I concealed carefully any need for people, cultivating an impression of independence. I turned tricks into real life, and real life into a sham. I found myself excluded from life on the inside as well as outside and was inevitably confounded by how or why people related to each other, seemingly so naturally"

(Williams, 2010, p. 37)

While infantile traumas are important as agents of suffering in adulthood, pathological developments are subjectively highly variable. The presence of psychopathological constructions, a disinclination for analytic dependence, and distortions of the superego can be counted among the factors that contribute to making some therapies especially arduous. We must also add that patients that are seriously ill do not approach analysis or any other type of therapy on their own account, perhaps because they are unaware of the level of their own suffering or because they fail to realise that treatment may work changes for the better. So, whoever decides to come into analysis has already achieved part of the journey.

With the analysis under way, what meaning does the adjective *difficult* hold, placed as it is before the noun *patient* and, thus, on the face of it negatively defining the analytic process? We could define as "difficult" all those patients showing reluctance to change during treatment or even those whose condition worsens. Traditionally, resistance to improvement, the analytic *impasse*, was thought to stem from the patient's own difficulties. Freud (1937c) himself believed that the patient boycotted any chance of recovery for fear of losing the secondary advantages afforded by his illness.

This idea has been overturned to an extent in recent decades: while possibly deriving from a particularly complex issue in the analysand, the impasse in therapeutic progress is now held to be mainly of an iatrogenic nature, owing to the analyst's partial inability to provide suitable responses to the patient's requests to evolve. When the analyst successfully tunes in to the patient's communications—which often pertain to the therapist's inadequate listening skills—the analytic process takes off again and further develops.

However, as I shall discuss in this chapter, another negative factor, stemming from the particular structure of the patient's psychopathology, often combines in many cases with the analyst's shortcomings in comprehension.

Clinical severity

We cannot automatically label "difficult" those patients who come to preliminary consultations with marked psychopathological symptoms, since the analytic outcome cannot be predicted merely on this basis. In other words, the gravity of the clinical symptomatology does not exclude *a priori* the patient from analysis; neither does it necessarily forecast an analytic course that will be more difficult than others or that will conclude negatively.

* * *

By way of illustration, many years ago a young female drug addict came to me for an analysis. I remember feeling very worried when I first met her. She arrived late for her first appointment, unkempt and dressed in black. Her face was expressionless, her voice monotonous, and she made no attempt at all to participate. With her slatternly appearance and way of talking, she resembled those long-term patients it was so common to see in psychiatric hospitals at the time.

She told me she had taken hard drugs for a long time and that she had been imprisoned for dealing, which she had done with her boyfriend. Her court case still had to be heard. She became an addict at a very young age. After failing to pass the high-school final exams, she decided to go to India, which was pretty common then, where she could take drugs freely.

I have to say that the first year of analysis, at five sessions a week, was extremely difficult for me. I was always afraid that my young analysand might succumb at any moment. In the past, she had injected large doses of heroin with the explicit aim of killing herself and her assertions now that she wanted to end her life sounded most convincing. In vain, she made sporadic attempts to stop, but her circle of friends was limited to young addicts of her age, and her boyfriend also continued to take drugs.

She generally arrived in analysis very late, sometimes only in the last five minutes. During the session, she frantically tried to gather her ideas together and to put some order into the events of the previous day that ended, almost always, in shooting up (usually heroin), followed sometimes by promiscuous sexual encounters.

For a year I managed to withstand the anxiety that the patient cascaded into me at every session. I did not know if or when she might be able to give up drugs. I only knew that I constantly had to come to terms with my anxiety and that I had to continue my analytic work without invading her with my demands.

Whenever it was possible I described the power that the drug held over her mind and her idealisation of death. There were many occasions when I would have liked to telephone her family and tell them to do something, perhaps get her admitted to hospital, but I never did.

On returning from the first summer holidays, after a year of analysis, she surprised me when she came into the session and said that she had stopped taking drugs. She had left her boyfriend and had succeeded in staying away from heroin. She added that she had had to do this during the holidays when she was far from me because only then could she be certain that it was her decision and that she had not done it just to please me.

From that moment, this young woman's life blossomed and flourished. She had only two relapses, for very short periods; both occurred subsequent to cancellation of the session—the first time I cancelled, the second she did. After much deliberation, she had decided to miss two sessions and go to visit a girlfriend who lived some distance away. On both occasions, she said, she had had to fall back on drugs to wipe out the intensely painful longing she felt for me in my absence.

*   *   *

If I had had to predict the outcome at the start of this analysis, bearing in mind the gravity of the situation, I would never have said it would be positive.

Thinking back over the patient's story as it emerged during the analytic treatment, I was able to pinpoint a number of elements that, with hindsight, threw light on the gap between the initial psychopathological picture and the positive outcome.

My young patient came from a family of well-off intellectuals. She had been considered somewhat retarded as a child as she did not excel at school, and so her parents had channelled all their expectations on to her younger brother. He had been sent to a child therapist for a time when experiencing a period of anxiety, but no one had noticed that my patient was a depressed little girl who withdrew into a fantasy world, which made it difficult for her to get on well at school.

Hence, my patient's sufferings clearly seemed linked to a disavowal of the self and to a very early relational trauma, while her recourse to drugs was a defence against the anxiety triggered by her feelings of non-existence, which had become unbearable as she approached her teenage years.

An emotionally sensitive type of listening on my part had given her the chance to emerge from her depression and stimulate her vital part. I had always sensed how important and profound her relationship with me was for her, right from the very start, and how useful and powerful the transference bond was for the good of the therapy.

In fact, as a baby, my young analysand must have enjoyed a certain amount of maternal warmth, as this type of affective receptiveness was soon reawakened in her in the transference. Although she was drug dependent, she was not destructive or cynical in her attitude to the world, or, in analysis, to me. Instead, she was deeply disappointed by her love objects and this had pushed her far from her affective relationships.

One of her first dreams clearly illustrated that she was aware that idealising drugs imprisoned her in a state close to death.

> In the dream, she was imprisoned in a Nazi concentration camp. She was going towards a building located in the centre of the camp in which a fantastically coloured and powerfully attractive insect lived, in a protected state. It was intensely seductive, and she fell prey to it. The dream clearly showed how her healthy part was aware of the danger stemming from her attraction to drugs (the beautiful insect) and so was asking for help to get out of its clutches.

Bearing in mind the therapeutic response, the case was not difficult. The analysis did not last long and concluded satisfactorily for both parties. Despite the presence of worrying symptoms, I believe that this patient was able to benefit from analytic treatment because her suffering stemmed from an infantile emotional trauma.

Although her parents had been mainly positive, they had not been capable of giving her an emotional place in their minds or of supporting her adequately as she grew older. This contributed to creating in her a feeling of futility and constant anxiety about falling into an existential void. Her healthy part, though suffering, had not been seriously breached and the pathological structures against emotional dependence were not very deeply rooted within her. In other words, the substantial, initial symptomatology did not mean that she became a difficult patient.

Pathogenic effects

Some patients who have had emotionally less receptive parents, as in the case above, are undoubtedly complex but not particularly difficult in analysis because, on the basis of a relationship with a new object, it is possible to help them reactivate the elements of emotional development that have remained paralysed.

On the other hand, other patients might not only have been deprived of an adequate emotional exchange but might also have incorporated their parents' mental states and anxieties. Particular emotional traumas—unusual even within the variation of mother–child relationships—can produce pathological distortions of considerable note.

While the intensity of the trauma can be equal, its effects can be different: much depends on the capacity of each individual to react and on the presence of a substitute figure (Modell, 1999).

In more complex situations, the child not only lacks a receptive object, but also suffers this same object intrusively projecting itself into his mind. Parents, at times, violate psychic boundaries and intrude with their anxieties or their delusional constructions, or they make their child a receptacle for their adult sexuality. In these cases, a link is generally created between the destabilising external situation and the mind that has to suffer it; early emotional traumas especially can inspire psychopathological structures that are destined to survive over time because they are perceived as supporting figures compared to the distressing experiences of dependence.

A deficiency of emotional containing, combined with the impossibility of projecting oneself into the other, results in these patients suffering psychophysical pain, confusion, and chronic anxiety. They often identify with the aggressor and their sense of self is constantly threatened with disintegration. Anger, due to frustration at parents particularly lacking in empathy, turns against the living part of the self, felt as a source of pain. A confused blend of expectations and disappointment is thus created that prompts feelings of emptiness and passivity.

In such cases, the crisis is accentuated when the patient begins to feel more alive and looks for an object capable of satisfying his needs but, never having had experience of one, he finds himself again full of anxiety and disoriented.

*   *   *

Thirty-seven-year-old Teresa[1] has been married for fifteen years and has a ten-year-old daughter.

A state of depression lasting several years with a concomitant abuse of alcohol—for which she was being treated by a psychiatrist who had prescribed a course of antidepressants—spurred her to come to analysis. She judged emblematic of the inadequacy of her mother the fact that, when she was small, she risked dying because her mother, who was breast-feeding her, did not realise that her milk was not nutritious enough. Instead, from infancy, she enjoyed a privileged, reciprocally idealising relationship with her father. This alliance was brusquely broken in adolescence.

Her first years at high school were marked by an increasing sense of inadequacy, constraint, and anger towards her parents, and isolation from her schoolmates. So, she became a heroin addict, which lasted for some years until she successfully detoxed after a period in rehabilitation.

During the early part of her analysis, Teresa continued to keep herself going with drink and with a singular inclination for pleasurable fantasies that detached her from the real world.

Towards her third year of analysis, when she had begun to feel better, Teresa became even more anxious. She felt very exposed and helpless; her nights were disturbed and she used to wake up full of anxiety. She was, in fact, afraid that without alcohol she would no longer be able to control her mind. Her only relief was provided by the fantasy of a uterus in which she found refuge. She felt like an invertebrate, spineless, exposed to any "mutation".

During this difficult stage of improvement, Teresa distanced herself from the analytic relationship and even missed a few sessions. Some weeks later, a dream helped her clarify the situation:

> "My husband and I, with our daughter, were in our house in the mountains, where we have a dog and a small cat. With the weekend over, we had to close up the house and leave food for the two animals that we couldn't take with us. We prepare bowls of food but realise that we cannot leave them there. So my husband and I decide to stay. I am overwhelmed by tremendous anxiety about the dark and about being alone. I sense my husband is suffering the same anxiety . . ."

Teresa speaks of the anxiety that torments her to such a degree at night that she is relieved to wake up in the morning and shrug off the pain. The dream vividly recalls her childhood anxiety when she was a little girl in bed in the dark: she would lie awake asking herself when her mother would return, dreading that no one would come back any more, feeling as though she would die, or would be squashed flat, or be split in half.

The animals in the dream and the anxiety appear to be linked to feeling herself alive: if she feels alive, she is frightened because immediately the risk of being left all alone emerges; there is no one to help, no one to think about her or look after her. It seems easier for her not to exist, to disappear in the general indifference and not to have any contact with her innermost needs and desires. The young animals undoubtedly stand for her vital desires and her anxiety stems from the sensation of not being able to succeed by herself, while not knowing who is capable of responding to her needs.

* * *

An object on which she can trustingly depend does not yet exist in this patient's mind; consequently, instead of heralding well-being, any improvement triggers fear and unbearable pain.

This situation recalls what Rosenfeld (1978) observes in the case of the baby who feels physical deprivation associated with a marked lack of maternal empathy. In this case, a confused blend of libido and destructive experiences lead to feelings of emptiness, weakness, and passivity that become a wish to die or to disappear into nothingness.

The solution adopted by Teresa was to kill her living parts. She probably adopted the same solution in early infancy when she found herself depending on a mother perceived as non-empathic and non-accepting. Paradoxically, her analytic improvement unleashes anxiety and entails the risk of a brusque step backwards.

Withdrawal

One of the most common outcomes of failed early emotional interaction sees the child withdrawing from human relationships to seek refuge in his own separate world. This dissociating from reality can occur either by way of full immersion in sensual and masturbatory self-stimulation or the creation of an imaginary world perceived as real. So the child becomes used to living in a secret *other world* that gives him pleasure. Steiner (1993) was the first to conceptualise the pathological structure of the *psychic retreat*.

I am convinced that this pathological structure can almost always be found in more complex, borderline, or psychotic patients. It is, in fact, a massive distortion in psychic functioning that hinders emotional development and growth and relationships.

In some cases, the child has to defend himself against being invaded by an adult (for example, a mother projecting her anxieties) by creating an inaccessible place in his mind; thus, the retreat would be the only space in which he can feel free and safe from adult intrusion. The combination of psychic deficiency and parental intrusion encourage the child to remain within his retreat, thus impeding him from experiencing emotional reality, which is constructed only on the basis of receptive exchanges with significant adults.

As I will explain later, the feeling of pleasure experienced in withdrawal is, for some patients, the real factor working against change.

The prolonged power and strength of this type of pathological structure stems from it having been established so early in the psyche and because the patient has no other way of functioning.

During analysis, the analysand can become aware of the pathological structure's ensnaring action, but his insight cannot create an opening towards the relational world until he has constructed other different internal objects to sustain him. In some cases, withdrawal seems to be the only feasible way out, as we can see with Teresa, fearful that too rapid an opening towards reality would obliterate her fantasy world, the only world possible for her to live in.

Symbolisation

The capacity for symbolising and attributing meaning to their own emotional states is damaged to a greater or lesser degree in difficult patients. Most probably, normal mother–child interaction, which is indispensable for structuring the self and for understanding one's emotional states, was not satisfactory in the experience of these patients. This fundamental emotional basis is organised before verbal language (Beebe et al., 1997).

Patients cannot develop an unconscious that makes use of symbolic language and that is capable of making emotional connections if these early emotional experiences are deficient. In fact, the system that—by way of repression—safeguards the conscious from the risk of being invaded by a chaotic excess of stimuli does not work in these patients.

Dependence

Patients who have not experienced good infantile dependence often mistrust all types of bond. To establish the necessary conditions for treatment, a protracted and circumspect approach must be adopted with them. For example, we must accept that the analysis will start at a reduced number of sessions with a view to being able to introduce a more suitable rhythm later on. However, some of these patients, despite all their initial declarations and behaviour, exhibit a profound attachment to the analyst figure once treatment has begun.

One of the reasons explaining this deep bond is that they are constantly tortured by confusional anxiety and paralysing doubts that lead them to perceive the analyst as a person capable of furnishing them with some direction—a skill in which they are lacking and of which they have great need.

Often, their confusion derives from being unable to distinguish between healthy objects and pathological objects, between aggression and destruction, between introjection and the anxiety to empty and destroy the object.

Confusional anxiety

Confusional anxiety in difficult patients varies in its nature. For the most part, it is an inability to distinguish between healthy and sick parts of the personality. The patient is usually dominated or seduced by a pathogenic structure that appears to be a guardian and source of energy and life, and in these cases will mistake excitement for real vitality. It might be necessary to work for a long time to help the patient re-establish in his internal world a distinction between exciting objects that do nothing to further growth and good objects that can also be frustrating. Another sort of confusion stems from being unable to distinguish between what is external and what belongs to the self. The patient often attributes blame or a negative meaning to normal, vital needs such as curiosity, desire, aggression, or passionate dependence.

*   *   *

As he began to improve, a borderline patient could not grasp the difference between the object's internalisation and its destruction. He had begun to feel a bond with me that continued after the sessions. Between one session and the next, he constantly thought of me and had the feeling that I was inside him. At the same time, he felt guilty and accused himself of literally possessing me: a voice had convinced him that he had cannibalistically swallowed me up. He was still unable to remember and perceive me as existing outside himself while at the same time being present within him. Another example of confusion between healthy objects and pathological ones is illustrated by a sexualised paedophile who tried to convince me that all children masturbate and that all adolescents have sex with each other (in actual fact he was talking about his early infancy spent in sexualised withdrawal; I discuss this patient further in Chapter Ten). Since he had not received a satisfactory response from me—in fact I had proffered a trite expression—he began to attack me in the next session because, in his eyes, I had materially become his sexualised part.

Pathological superego

While it is always important to explore the structure of the superego, it is especially important to do so with difficult patients, as they often harbour a well-entrenched pathological superego that has lost its stabilising function and arouses accusations or feelings of persecutory guilt. Green (2011) believes that some patients can be considered "difficult" because they suffer from the excessive burden of a very severe, paralysing superego that configures a regressive form of masochism.

These patients are tormented by guilt directed not necessarily at their aggressiveness, but more often at blaming their desires or affective needs. They appear to have internalised an object that blames need and that, most probably, reproduces the same reproachful response with which their mother might originally have greeted their attempts at emotional closeness.

Emotional dependence is considered a sign of weakness or failure. Hence, the superego attacks whatever is good and useful for development. Consequently, the superego that has installed itself in the internal world of these patients has both severe and cruel sides to it and seems to instigate deadly and anti-vital behaviour. In other cases, the superego appears as a destabilising and confusing agent, driving the patient to a state of mental arrogance and exaltation before casting him down into a state of guilt that is impossible to repair. This is why our first task with difficult patients is to interpret the superego's structure in order to isolate and contain it, since otherwise all subsequent analytic communications will be distorted.

Some traumatised patients, whose mothers probably rejected their attempts at closeness, at the same time making them feel guilty about it, show a particular form of confusion between a desire for relationships and invasiveness.

* * *

This can be exemplified by a patient whose female analyst, who had recently moved her studio closer to where she lived, had informed the patient that she would have to reduce the number of sessions a week from four to three in the following three months. Since the patient made no comment, the analyst attempted to explore her feelings on this point. The patient said that she was not displeased about the analyst's decision; in fact, she felt relieved. She appreciated the fact that the analyst knew how to safeguard her own private space, unlike her mother, who worked tirelessly all day long, even when it was not necessary, but complained about it constantly. In addition, the fact that the analyst had just moved her studio closer to her home might arouse in the patient a desire for greater intimacy, proof of her invasiveness that would certainly have disturbed the analyst.

* * *

What is good in this case, the intimacy and desire for a relationship, is regarded as negative.

In other cases, what is destructive is idealised and held as a goal to be pursued. This type of confusion is present in anorexia, where the patient refuses to acknowledge that his anorexic behaviour can lead to death. Since denying oneself food is an extraordinary experience, the anorexic is oblivious to the fact that being attracted to this mental state is tantamount to being attracted to death. Sometimes, this attraction to death is revealed; for example, in dreams featuring a wonderful landscape in which a graveyard is especially beautiful or brightly coloured.

> Traumatised in infancy, a patient of mine dreamt—during a particularly sad and difficult time in her life and her analysis—of flying over a small village set in a stunning Mediterranean landscape and perched high above the blue sea, and of wanting to dive into the water. The seaside village was associated to the Greek island on which the patient's father, together with other Italian officers, had been shot during the war and thrown into the sea by German soldiers.

These mental states and dreams are characterised by an absence of anxiety, which, together with the idealisation of death, allows self-destruction to gain a hold. It is vital that the analyst's interpretation in these cases, which also present constant fluctuations between withdrawal and a search for relationships, between states of excitement and depression, is always extremely accurate and specific for the type of mental functioning it is addressing.

Sometimes, the patient's confusional state and underlying persecutory anxieties result in a distorted understanding of the analyst's communications, which are then inserted into the patient's particular vision of the world. To avoid misunderstanding, it is essential that the analyst's responses not only reflect the patient's communication but also bear in mind his point of view; the risk is that even apparently obvious analytic responses might not be so for the patient and thus trigger further confusional anxiety. As a result, the patient often feels attacked and, in turn, reacts by attacking the analyst.

Rather than interpreting eventual personal or transference conflicts in these cases, it is more effective to describe to the patient how his mind is functioning, as is apparent from his dreams and communications, so that he can gradually begin to comprehend himself. The analyst must also know the world—made up of beliefs, convictions, and falsifications that are not perceived as such—that these patients inhabit and in which they have enclosed themselves. Similarly, the analyst must have a full grasp of what the patient is capable or incapable of understanding and the context into which the patient will insert and eventually distort his interpretations. This prevents impasses arising that might interfere with the course of the analysis.

Psychic withdrawal, dependence denial, superego distortion, and confusion between objects and functions are the primary pathogenic nuclei that, in my opinion, lie at the root of the pathologies of difficult cases.

These pathogenic configurations are so old and well embedded that it is difficult to completely sever their power over the patient. However, even if the pathological structures have not quite disappeared by the end of analysis, new horizons have opened up and new objects coexist alongside the old ones. While the patient returning to old pathologies cannot be excluded, it does mean that he can, at the same time, keep open new paths that he has developed during treatment.

By way of example, I recall a patient who had been precociously withdrawn in a masturbatory world as a child. Before coming to analysis, as an adult, he lived in a world dissociated from reality, totally immersed in pornographic websites and sexualised fantasies.

* * *

After many years of therapy, which had led to great improvement, it seemed as though the time had come to end the analysis. After working through this event with the patient for a long time, the analysis was concluded. However, I was not entirely comfortable with this decision: the very early origin and profound roots of the patient's sexualised withdrawal, together with the fact that the old seduction still sporadically appeared in his dreams, left me with lingering doubts as to whether it was the right decision. On the other hand, I was convinced that I had given him all the possible wherewithal and that considerable changes had been made in the course of his long therapy.

A year and a half later he telephoned me and asked to see me. I confess that I had had some doubts as to his ability not to fall back into old ways and thought he wanted to ask for some supplementary analysis. When I saw him, I immediately realised I was wrong. He was happy and seemed younger and better looking. He had lost a lot of weight that had previously made him look a little awkward. He spoke about his analysis as a highly significant experience and was moved on recalling it.

At the end of the meeting I said he looked thinner and asked him how he'd done it. He replied, "Yes, it's true, doctor, and so simple. Just don't look at food. It's a bit like with pornography, if I don't look at it, I don't feel tempted."

* * *

In these preliminary pages, I have illustrated a number of constellations that we often find in difficult patients. A characterising aspect is that they require long analyses, primarily because the pathogenic constellations are so strongly embedded in their personality in such a structured way and at such an early date. Hence, the work of dismantling and reconstructing the identity requires much constant effort on the part of both analyst and analysand. This is the case for certain patients, for example perverse ones, who organised their withdrawal at a very early age; we are certainly on difficult terrain with them, although it is relatively predictable.

However, it is not the case for borderline or psychotic patients, who I will discuss in the final chapters of this book. They present an entirely different psychic context. Just as physicists cannot adopt traditional physics for studying the atom, so we analysts cannot use the psychoanalytic method created for understanding neurotic patients to approach the world of psychotics. There is a decided difference in quality between the neurotic and the psychotic context.

I believe that in both borderline and psychotic states, something vitally important for psychic survival was lost in infancy. In borderline patients, this lack of maternal empathy, together with emotional traumas, might have impeded the psychic function capable of containing emotions.

Consequently, these patients are incapable of reacting in an effective and fitting way to constant normal environmental frustrations. They lack emotional competency and might short-circuit explosively at any moment. As a result, they find it difficult to learn from the experience and their analytic journey is very arduous.

While it is relatively easy to identify what might have been past environmental traumas in borderline patients, these traumas are not so evident or easily identifiable in psychotic patients. In fact, it would seem that even as small children these patients were attracted to a dissociated world of mental functioning that, over time, has produced the psychopathological constructions (the delusions and hallucinations) that characterise the evolution of the illness. The specific nature of psychosis means that once the pathological change has occurred, it is obstinately tenacious. These cases reveal a constant struggle between the psychotic part that does not want to relinquish its hold and the healthy part that asks to be sustained and reinforced so that it can contain the sick part.

I have already mentioned that psychotic transformation tends to be irreversible. It must be kept under careful observation during therapy and we must accept the fact that *generally*, throughout the analytic process of psychotic states, the delusion will continue to appear. Just like Freud, who first believed transference to be a drawback of the treatment but then embraced it as the keystone of therapy, so, too, we must think of the delusion as a normal event that can tell us much about how to treat our patient.

Furthermore, we must not forget that today we work in decidedly more favourable conditions than in the past, as we have recourse to the use of medicines for containing the most acute and dangerous moments of psychotic manifestations.

In challenging our models and theories, difficult patients compel us to question ourselves about the efficacy of our clinical and theoretical apparatus.

I use the word *difficult* in this book and not *serious* because, as I have already mentioned, the gravity of a patient's symptoms does not necessarily herald an unsatisfactory outcome. The clinical complexity of difficult cases constantly challenges our analytic insight. In other words, I believe that the treatment of these patients provides us with a valuable incentive to greater exploration and knowledge of the pathological distortions of the human mind and to an attentive assessment of its powers for reparation.

CHAPTER TWO

Trauma as a source of pathology

"'Eternal rehabilitation from a trauma of unknown nature':
where did the beautiful title of your book come from?"
Andrea Zanzotto: "I was referring to the concept of life in the
broadest sense"

(Zanzotto, 2007, p. 16, translated for this edition)

In psychoanalysis, the concept of trauma has had a chequered
history, both in terms of its definition and of the importance attributed to it as a cause of illness in adults. In the past, a single, unexpected, and violent event was considered traumatic. After Khan (1963)
introduced the concept of cumulative trauma, psychoanalysts also
turned their attention to the pathogenic elements involved in the
distortion of the mother–child emotional relationship. In the case of
difficult patients, many events, even if they are not particularly violent, are considered sources of future pathology because they cause a
violation of the child's psychic apparatus.

The extent to which trauma effects the development of psychopathology is a controversial subject. Some analysts, in fact, seem to
believe that the suffering afflicting patients stems from their imaginary

life rather than from their "real" life. While discussing the uncertainty reigning in psychoanalytical circles about this point, Bollas (1995, p. 103) writes,

> The psychoanalytical insistence on the priority of the imagined—juxtaposed, if necessary, to the happened—is understandable, if regrettable. Each person's inclination to describe his present state of the mind as determined by external events is countered by the psychoanalytic perspective, which insists that such an account must be regarded in terms of the person's potential wishes or object-relational aims, even if it coincides with events which have, so to speak, happened. Do we have to choose between the imagined and the happened? Are they opposed?

This quandary had engaged Freud, too; at the start, he had believed that sexual trauma was the origin of hysteria but, subsequently, had retraced his steps and established that his patients modified their memories of the past. From that moment, he emphasised the importance of the psychic reality, the internal world constructed by the subject, thus shifting the pathogenic effects of the real trauma into a secondary position. Many authors after him followed the trend that privileges internal over external reality; others, instead, set out in a different direction. This has resulted in a complex mesh of observations and diverse and, at times, contradictory hypotheses.

In an attempt to clarify the multiple analytical approaches to trauma and to its pathogenic role, I will describe the various contributions made, up to the most recent, in chronological order.

Trauma and Freud

Freud explored the traumatic event in various ways. Since a *sexual trauma* always emerged in his patients' childhood stories, he at first believed that the origin of the neurosis was of a traumatic nature; the pathogenic effect of the childhood trauma did not depend so much on its disturbing effect as on the activation of a series of unconscious excitations of a sexual nature. Thus, in his original view, the trauma does not produce immediate consequences; its effects are manifested at the onset of adult sexuality because the conflict emerges only in that moment of activation. The anxiety expresses the conflict between sexual desire, empowered by the childhood erotic experience, and denial of it owing to it being repressed.

Freud did not consider the intrusion of adult sexuality into the infant psyche to be a disturbing element, but believed that stimulation of sexual desire was important. It must be pointed out that in this period Freud had not yet formulated his concept of psychosexuality (something he would do in 1905) and regards sexuality as akin to sexual desire.

In the case of Dora, Freud (1905e) attempted to make the patient aware of how she had been aroused by Mr K's sexual proposals. He hoped that Dora would confirm his theory that the illness resulted from the posthumous action of a sexually exciting trauma. The patient's symptom of nausea corresponded to the sexual arousal shifting from the genitals to the mouth in an unconscious desire for oral relations. Freud had formulated the hypothesis that Dora was unconsciously in love with Mr K and repressed the resulting sexual arousal, without bearing in mind that a fourteen-year-old girl might have felt disturbed by the sexual intrusion of an adult. A significant example of Freud's constant misunderstandings of the patient's communications is the dream with which Dora abandons analysis: she wanders about in a square in which a monument to a famous man stands (one presumes it is Freud), but does not go to the dead father's funeral (the analyst dies without her feeling any regrets at all).

After abandoning the aetiological hypothesis of sexual trauma, we know Freud sustained that anxiety was triggered not so much by the real trauma but by the *fantasy of seduction*.

The childhood suffering of young Hans (Freud, 1909b) in fact had nothing to do with any traumatic event. A young child with good parents, Hans lived in an apparently calm and tranquil middle-class environment. The trauma had occurred in his internal world, owing to a conflict between instinctual forces and fear of punishment: the horse that terrified him was the traumatising image of a castrating father who wanted to punish him for his oedipal desires.

The effect the real trauma has on the psyche returned once more to centre stage when Freud, during the First World War, had to study the effects of the traumas of war. This led to his profound insights into the significance of the traumatic impact on the psyche.

In *Beyond the Pleasure Principle*, Freud (1920g) had used the word "trauma" in a descriptive way, imagining the mind enclosed within a *protective membrane*, a barrier against excessive stimuli, which can be pierced by a wound. In *Inhibitions, Symptoms and Anxiety* (1926d), he had described a number of basic traumas, such as love from significant objects suddenly ending, maternal deprivation, and also loss of the superego's protection. For example, in melancholia the patient loses the love of the superego, which becomes a critical agent.

Pathogenic effects of trauma

Psychic trauma is a sudden or repeated action that proves to be *damaging because the necessary protective defences are not yet ready* to deal with such an overwhelming blow that cannot be understood or worked through. Traumas producing catastrophic effects occur at every age, but not all traumatic events produce damage. Indeed, the pathogenic effect of an event depends not only on its intensity, but also on the age and stage of development of the individual who suffers it. What might be pathological at one age might not be so in a subsequent period. Furthermore, we must bear in mind that an isolated event might not always have a pathogenic effect, since an individual's natural repairing capacity can lessen the damage.

I have already mentioned the protective membrane of the psyche, which can be lacerated by trauma. For newborns and small babies, the protective filter is exercised by the mother on the basis of her spontaneous capacity to intuit what the child is capable of enduring in the various moments of its emotional development.

Among pathogenic effects resulting from trauma, we must distinguish the acute and immediate ones from the insidious ones that take time to emerge. We can postulate a scale for early traumas that ranges from cases in which emotional development is totally destroyed (in these cases the traumatic experience is not representable because it occurred before the capacity to understand psychic facts) to situations in which partial damage occurs (as in childhood sexual traumas that lead to partial inhibition of emotional development).

Current psychiatric nosography places the effects of traumatic events in the post traumatic stress disorder (PTSD) syndrome. One of the characteristics of this syndrome is constant repetition of the traumatic event: instead of being forgotten, the disagreeable event is constantly repeated. To annul the anxiety threatening it, the mental apparatus creates a dissociation in the conscious state: the trauma is deleted in a normal conscious state but can emerge unexpectedly from the dissociated conscious state.

Environmental trauma

The concept of the protective membrane, formulated by Freud within the economic concept of the psychic apparatus, was subsequently enriched by authors who emphasised the importance of the infant's first emotional experiences and of environmental interferences.

Among these, Ferenczi (1955[1933]) highlighted the ways in which a child's sensitivity and competence can be endangered by adults when the latter intrude with their own needs into his private area.

Balint (1968), a Hungarian analyst and follower of Ferenczi, speaks of the *basic fault*, something that occurs in the earliest months of life and that leads to a lack of integration between mother and child; the traumatic breaches derive from the mother's incapacity to adapt to the basic needs of her baby.

Similar to infant rheumatic fever, which produces damage that appears only later in adult life, so, too, the effects of emotional trauma are manifested in an unpredictable way and in later years. The function of the protective membrane of the mind corresponds to the parents' emotional competence in intuitively knowing what psychic experiences their child is capable of tolerating.

In Winnicott's "dual mother–child unit" (1971) and in Bion's "container–contained" (1970), the mother represents the barrier against an excess of stimuli. Prolonged trauma results from a failed maternal function of containing and, in extreme cases, from the parents' projections of their pathological psychic contents into the child's mind. This type of trauma is clearly expressed in the concept of *cumulative trauma* proposed by Khan (1963), who coherently applies Winnicott's intuition when he describes a child that needs its mother and a mother that is part of the child's self. In the case of cumulative trauma, the child responds to its mother's repeated intrusions with inhibitions or distortions in his psychological development.

In the earliest period in life, traumatic experiences are not memorised because memories are established only when there is a capacity for representing and understanding the significance of an event. Joseph and Anne-Marie Sandler (1987) postulate the existence of an *unconscious past*, made up of a series of events of which one is unaware and that are impossible to recover, and of an *unconscious present*, which is accessible and which is formed later on the basis of representable emotional experiences. Only the latter can be repressed and forgotten; in other words, it can be rendered unconscious, although available for future recovery.

The Sandlers' intuitions have been confirmed by current work undertaken in the field of the neurosciences that distinguishes an *explicit memory* and an *implicit one*. Explicit memory allows intentional remembering of a forgotten event, while implicit memory refers to something that has been learnt but which is impossible to make conscious; these are events or processes that occurred precociously, before the capacity for representation was developed. The theory posits that the precursors of thought and affectivity, which are formed through unaware processes, can be disturbed in the very first months by traumatic events.

Following this line of thought, Fonagy (1999) postulates that the borderline states derive from precocious traumas, incorporated before the possibility for representing them existed. Borderline and psychotic patients would, therefore, be incapable of mentalising, or, rather, of representing the emotions, psychic events, and mental states whose meaning they are unaware of.

Consequently, we can better appreciate Balint, who intuited that precocious trauma is incorporated in the structure of the ego itself and leads to its malfunctioning.

On reviewing the concept of dissociation, the most recent works on the effects of sexual trauma (Davies, 1996) shine new light on Breuer's contribution about the mechanism at work in his hysterical patients. Breuer did not agree with Freud about the importance of repression, but instead stressed a vertical dissociation in the conscious state. Repression is a process by which an experience relegated to the unconscious cannot be spontaneously remembered but can be recovered once the obstacle that censured it is overcome. Dissociation is a more radical process that not only refers to awareness, but also interests the conscious state. With dissociation, memory of the abuse is dissociated and, when it emerges, it has the quality of a dream, as though it did not belong to the subject's experience.

From a certain point of view, we can say that Breuer's proposal of the concept of dissociation in the oneiroid states of hysteria (the second condition)—derived from Janet—was more accurate. In Freud's mind, instead, repression was the main defence in his model of the general functioning of the unconscious. But if we look at the dynamics of the serious psychopathologies, as suffered by the hysterical patients who came to analysis in Freud's time, we have to acknowledge that Breuer's proposal fitted the psychopathological picture better.

Indeed, dissociation occurs when it is not possible to use repression: in other words, when the level of anxiety is so high that it must be dissociated; a part of the mind itself is dissociated—traumatic memory—which becomes inaccessible. Dissociation is considered the specific result of an unbearable trauma.

The contribution made by the neurosciences

Neuroscientists have provided assistance in understanding how traumatic memories are dissociated. As mentioned earlier, they tell us that man has two distinct memories that work in parallel: the *explicit* or *declarative* memory and the *implicit* or *procedural* one.

To clarify: an example of explicit memory is the memory of the place in which a person married. Procedural memory, instead, corresponds to an acquired skill, such as how to ride a bicycle, or to an automatic behaviour, such as an immediate reaction to a shock. Declarative memory is permeable and allows an event to be recalled by willpower, whereas procedural memory is impermeable to recall.

The difference between explicit and implicit memory was discerned while observing a patient suffering from a serious form of epilepsy: large parts of the patient's parietal lobes had been removed. After the operation, the patient lost his capacity to remember the past, but, although completely incapable of pinpointing events, was able to acquire new motor skills even if he could not remember when and how he had learnt them (Scoville & Milner, 1957).

The two memories have two different cerebral systems, distinct both from a development point of view and from an anatomical one. Explicit memory depends on the function of the hippocampus, whose bilateral destruction results in losing the possibility of memorising an event. The emotional component, especially fear and anxiety, is, instead, recorded in the amygdala.[2] Implicit memory depends on the basal ganglia and the cerebellum (Levin, 2009). This neurophysiological structuring of memory allows us to understand what happens on impact with the traumatic event.

Traumatic memories are codified by the brain in different ways from everyday memories. LeDoux (1996) postulates that memories of fear are branded on the mind due to excitement of the amygdala function. Indeed, the amygdala is part of the primitive circuit of fear that has little connection with the cortical circuit, where the more complex functions of integration and elaboration of psychic experiences take place. The amygdala records the trauma that remains incorporated in the primitive circuit, where it cannot be transformed.

The explanation advanced by some neuroscientists (Jacobs & Nadel, 1985) about why memory of the event (the province of the hippocampus) is disconnected from its emotional memory (recorded in the amygdala) postulates that, during the traumatic event, an excess of hydrocortisone (in its turn stimulated by the adrenalin produced in conditions of stress) is produced that annihilates the function of the hippocampus, so increasing the role of the amygdala. Consequently, conscious memory is weak, if not absent, while the emotional memory of the traumatic event remains extremely vivid and is reactivated in the presence of a stimulus connected to the trauma.

For example, a person who has survived a railway crash might have panic attacks every time he sees fog outside his window. This is because he unconsciously associates fog with the billowing smoke produced during the crash.

Sexual abuse

Theorising trauma and the dissociated state is a recent rediscovery of psychoanalysis. The concept of dissociation re-emerged when a number of serious psychopathological states (Vietnam veterans with post-trauma syndromes and victims of sexual abuse) were studied.

According to modern psychoanalytic views, from Bion onwards, repression is not only a defence, but also a mechanism that allows the experience lived to become unconscious. Without repression, the emotional contents would remain in the conscious and could never be dreamt or transformed into thought.

Dissociation, instead, intervenes when repression is no longer sufficient; that is, when the level of anxiety is so great that the event must be dissociated. Whatever is dissociated becomes a part of the mind itself, the traumatic memory, which is no longer accessible.

I would like to point out that a concept very similar to dissociation was described by Freud in the later years of his work when he spoke of denial; in other words, an operation that does not want to recognise perceptions of reality. But in this context, we are dealing with splitting and not dissociation. An analogous process was described by Melanie Klein in splitting and projection; this, too, is part of the normal defence mechanisms, but becomes pathological if used excessively.

I would like to recall the pioneering research of Selma Fraiberg (1982) that highlighted the pathological dissociative defences of early childhood, and her work on ghosts in the nursery, in which she points to the intergenerational transmission of trauma. I would also like to mention Bowlby's attachment theory, and the most recent studies on disorganised attachment, in which children fall into trance-like or self-hypnotic states.

For a decade or so now, and thanks principally to the contribution of North American authors, the question of traumatic memories has been brought to our attention again, and especially the memories of emotional traumas created when a love object, for example, a parent, uses his child as a sexual object.

Yovell (2000) describes how the emotional memory of the trauma emerged in the therapy of a patient who had been regularly abused when only four years old by a young family friend. As well as eating disorders and constant depression, Tara (the name of the young patient) had developed an emotional inhibition that prevented her from having a significant relationship with a man. During therapy, she had become more open to relationships and had met someone she liked.

*   *   *

After spending an evening with this person in her home, during which an increasingly intimate situation had been created, Tara returned to the session the next day very depressed and anxious and said that as soon as this young man had left she had felt an urgent need to run to the bathroom and wash herself and had had to stuff herself with food, something that had not happened for months. She had also had a terrible dream that had woken her up and prevented her from going back to sleep. In the dream she saw herself as a child playing in the garden with her playmates. At a certain point a huge snake appeared in the grass: at the beginning it was friendly and brightly coloured, and cheerfully slithered between the young girls' legs. Then it began to coil itself tightly around Tara until she felt she might suffocate. Terrified, she looked around her and saw that all her friends were dead. In the second part of the dream, Tara moved towards the house and went into the kitchen where she glimpsed her mother, from behind, trying desperately to hack the snake into pieces and so make it disappear. Her mother noticed the little girl and stared at her with hatred as though she had uncovered a secret.

*   *   *

Listening to the dream, Yovell began to think that the intimacies exchanged with her boyfriend the night before (they had passionately kissed) had triggered the dissociated memory of an abuse. For this reason, Tara had felt terribly anxious and guilty when the young man had gone home. Talking about it with her brother some time later, Tara discovered that she had been abused in infancy by a neighbour who used to play with them, but the family had decided not to talk about it with her. The dream had reawakened in Tara the original trauma of being forced to succumb to an all-enveloping and penetrating snake-penis. It is important to point out that the dream also showed her awareness of her mother's knowledge of the abuse that she (mother) continued to keep secret.

Traumatic anxiety, relating back to an experience of impotence and terror endured alone, is not *thinkable* and must be denied. However, it remains alive in the dissociated memory and cannot be forgotten. For an event to be forgotten, it has to be made work-through-able, transformable, and digestible by our mind. Only what can be *digested* can be forgotten, like dreams that serve to integrate our thoughts and which are then forgotten.

Pathogenic effects having similar characteristics

In works dealing with sexual abuse, the defensive aspects that lead to dissociating the trauma from the conscious state are generally emphasised, as exemplified by the case of Tara above. The development of the psychopathological structures that can be generated as a consequence of sexual abuse is, however, less frequently described.

I remember a patient abused by her father; whenever there was a crisis in the analytic relationship, she got herself into sexually promiscuous situations or mentally excited states that were often described in dreams. In so doing, the patient seemed to be repeating the difficult relationship with her mother, from whom she had distanced herself in childhood to merge erotically with her father. This preference for her father led to a definitive break with the maternal figure and had increased the child's narcissism.

Children abused by psychotic mothers tend to sexually seduce the analyst during therapy quite openly. This event would confirm Freud's early hypothesis that sexual abuse can trigger unconscious arousal of a sexual nature in the child.

Abraham (1973[1907]) was the first to describe the process of sexualisation that can follow on from sexual trauma. Observing that sexual abuse is more frequently encountered in sick, hysterical, or psychotic people, Abraham postulated that some children arrive precociously at sexual pleasure and, because of this, can associate with adult abusers without adopting excessive defences. The precocious encounter with sexuality indicates that disruptive elements of development are already at work. Abraham thus proposed an overturned sequence in which sexual withdrawal precedes the trauma and encourages it. The trauma would not be the *primum movens* of the psychopathological development, but the symptom of an already abnormal situation. For Abraham, child sexual trauma does not play an aetiological role in hysteria and psychosis, but, instead, expresses a predisposition in childhood to the subsequent neurosis or psychosis.

CHAPTER THREE

Trauma in the primary relationship

"The idea of trauma involves a consideration of external factors; in other words it belongs to dependence. Trauma is a failure relative to dependence"

(Winnicott, 1989, p. 145)

T he life stories of difficult patients are interlaced with traumatic infantile experiences that cannot be disregarded in our analytic work because the traumatic event constantly resurfaces, not only in their anxieties and in the transference, but also in their dreams. This is why the analyst must keep the emotionally disturbing environment in mind so that he can prepare an appropriate emotional setting for each specific story. The direct effects of the traumatic experience and, above all, its indirect effects—in other words, the aggregate of individual responses in the form of psychopathological structures that were triggered by the trauma—determine the clinical problem.

In "Analysis terminable and interminable" (1937c) Freud states that analysis, even if successfully concluded, cannot prevent eventual relapses from recurring and that an interminable analysis would be required to satisfactorily tackle all the situations a patient will experience throughout his life.

So how can the analyst help the patient escape his preordained lot?

If we proffer only knowledge during the patient's treatment, we would merely be playing out the role of the chorus in Greek tragedy. The chorus knows the whole story but limits itself to reporting events and commenting on what happens to the protagonist, who, in spite of everything, hastens to meet his fate. His tragedy is played out without the chorus making any attempts to modify it (Brenman, 2002).

Tragedy in the past

Bollas (1989) highlights an interesting distinction between *destiny* and *fate*. The word *destiny* indicates the potential course of a person's life and corresponds to his specific nature, or unique set of peculiarities (which the author calls *idiom*): an unconscious preconception inscribed in each person that urges him to realise his creative potential. Yet, *fate* implies not being free and true to oneself, but constrained by life's events and story. A person can shape his own destiny if he is fortunate, determined, and sufficiently aggressive. For Bollas, this will depend on the protagonist's action and drive, whereas fate is revealed through the words of the gods announced by oracles (as for Oedipus).

Being unable to imagine a future is a particular type of loss that causes the individual to remain arrested in endless repetitions of which he is quite unaware. The person who comes to analysis can be described as an individual struck by fate who has no sense of his own future, and it is this specific element that fuels his anxiety.

Independently of whether we choose to pursue a trauma theory or an intrapsychic theory to aid understanding of our analysand's suffering, I think we must all agree that the tragedy has already occurred in every patient we encounter and whom we would like to help. The past has already created the basis for the age-old destiny to be repeated and that is why we, quite apart from all our excellent theories and in-depth clinical experience, can always be relegated to the role of the Greek chorus. We must avoid a unilateral vision of infancy and keep well to the fore all the variables that interfere with development. These are determined not only by eventually insufficient or distorted responses of the primary objects, but also by the child's subjective inclination to create defences or psychopathological structures that increase in importance over time.

Trauma in the primary relationship

Green gives us a very effective illustration of emotional trauma in his classic essay "The dead mother" (2001), in which he analyses the effect of maternal depression on the child. He concludes that, even if the mother is physically present, her mental absence implies psychic catastrophe for the child. In these cases, the child frequently identifies with the mother and, subsequent to her massive and radical withdrawal, forms a psychic hole in place of the absent object. Loss of love is followed by loss of meaning: a sense of self does not in fact develop unless nurtured by maternal empathy. Following this line of thought, Green sees a close link between the individual traumatic infantile experience and the development of psychopathology in the adult.

Modell (1999) distinguishes the single traumatic experience (such as, for example, the one described by Freud in the case of the Wolf Man) from the accumulation of emotional experiences resulting from a constant lack of maternal participation. He points out that infant research has confirmed that, by the age of ten months, the emotional response of babies of depressed mothers is already organised differently from that of babies of normal mothers (Beebe et al., 1997; Tronick, 1989). While emphasising the specific characteristics of individual development (even the brains of homozygotic twins differ both structurally and functionally), Modell believes that a countless number of decisive elements contributes to the pathological consequences of a developmental process and that a selective factor determines the effect of a specific environmental trauma. For example, the exuberant nature of a child or the willingness of a maternal substitute to take care of him will be crucial in determining his response to the trauma.

By *emotional trauma* or *trauma in the primary relationship*, I mean the aggregate of distorted responses that are capable of conditioning the child's development in a psychopathological sense. Clinical experience confirms the traumatic effect of early distortions of *emotional communication* between the parents' minds and the child's mind. What is at stake in the case of difficult patients is not so much the emotional absence of the primary object, but the intrusion of that object's sick,

superego, or distorted parts (Williams, 2004). And so we find ourselves dealing with an internalised object that behaves as though it
was part of the patient; in the more complex pathologies, these introjections work against the patient, at times seducing him, at others
intimidating him, but always confusing him.

Williams believes that a pathological parent can invade the child's
mind in order to get rid of excited or frankly sick parts of himself that
he cannot hold within himself. In this way, the child becomes a
container for these sick parts and loses all perception of being a separate person. Once identification with the sick parent has occurred, the
patient senses the invasive object within him and at the same time
feels he has been invaded by alien and incomprehensible objects. It is
as though the patient absorbs and identifies with an excited or
psychotic part of the parent that is perceived as part of the self and
that at the same time creates confusion between the self and the other.
The following clinical case seems to me to be highly pertinent.

> Laura is twenty-three years old, obtained her school diploma, lives at
> home but supports herself with a part-time job in a hotel.[3]

> She is very late for the first meeting, having realised the correct the time
> of the appointment much too late. She seems very anxious and confused.
> She does not know where to begin, but after a bit of hesitation starts to
> talk about her relationship with her father, which makes her very uncom-
> fortable and which she calls "incestuous". Only he and her paternal
> grandmother had any say in her education, while her mother was seem-
> ingly distant and a marginal figure. Retired and a heavy drinker, her
> father likes to take her with him when he goes out socially, excluding her
> mother who, in his words, he would have liked to exchange when she got
> to forty with two women of twenty.

> Laura says she has rather a problem with alcohol: she drinks a bit too
> much wine and at night drinks spirits to help her get to sleep. At home, it
> is often her father who encourages her to drink, acting a bit like a dealer
> with an addict who wants to quit. She has no stable emotional relation-
> ship. She always responds to whoever seems interested in having a sexual
> fling with her, but these relationships never lead anywhere. In fact, she
> does not really know whether she prefers women or men.

> Her emotional sphere seems to have been, and still is, very disturbed by
> the presence of her father. Laura says that he has always criticised her,
> while at the same time constantly intruding: "Even the other evening he

asked me if I wanted to go out for a smoke and a chat, but now I ask myself why on earth it is necessary, with all the time there is for chatting, to always have to create these twosome situations. At home I'm tense; I can't stand him always needling me, smothering me with kisses, pinching me, running his hands through my hair or touching my ears to show his affection. If I push him away, he's hurt and I feel guilty."

Laura starts analysis at three sessions a week and from the very beginning shows a strong attachment to the analyst. During the first months she often describes a confused existential picture that lacks any significance: she looks for a new job, full of anxiety and with little success; she tries to put a bit of order into her life, again unsuccessfully. Extremely confused moments emerge in her emotional life. To escape her anxiety and the paternal invasion she goes out and meets up with some acquaintances, with whom she ends up in bed.

Importantly, she attempts to bring into analysis—so that she can escape its hold over her—a confusing internal object connected to her experience with her father. This internal object is two-faced: one, belittling; the other, arousing.

A critical point appears in a dream soon after resuming sessions following the first Christmas break: "I had to come to the session but I knew I was late, so I asked my father to take me to Milan. While we were driving here he kept on shouting at me because I forget everything; I looked at my watch and saw that the time was almost up, so I said that I wanted to come just for the last five minutes to explain how stupid I am, but I suddenly realised I'd got the day wrong too."

A second dream reveals the arousing and dangerous aspect of the invasive paternal object: "I had a nightmare tonight. Once I'd got back home, my father came up to me and started his customary caresses but I was less uptight than usual and made him understand that they upset me. The usual things, his hands in my hair and ears, kisses on my neck and so on. Then I went to bed and had this dream: I was in bed and the bed was in the position it used to be in when I slept with one eye open, up until the time I had a sort of breakdown and fainted and my parents wanted to take me to hospital. My father was there, touching me more urgently than he did really and calling me Ariel; I wanted to scream but got a hold of myself and told myself not to as it was only a dream and so I woke up, but it took me quite a long time to work out exactly where I was and to understand the position the bed was in . . ." The patient associates to the period in which she could not sleep and was extremely anxious, and perhaps even persecuted, to the extent of risking psychiatric hospitalisation. Her anxiety also appears to be connected to the intrusion of this arousing paternal object that manipulates her mind until she becomes Ariel, a pure angelic spirit. This picture plainly portrays a risk of slipping towards a psychotic transformation.

I have included this case because I believe it clearly illustrates how this patient's inner world risks possible transformation as a result of unremitting emotional trauma. Laura was incapable of producing antibodies against the trauma and was, instead, colonised. Without being aware of this, she is prey to an invasive object that confuses and arouses her. While her father's conduct is highly disturbing, it is also true that Laura has made this invasive internal object her own—it has become part of her—and that she looks on it as a sort of cure. In the dream in which Laura is deeply anxious, the arousal procured by this object is visualised as highly pathogenic. This point marked the beginning of the patient's awareness of the deadly nature of the invasive object.

From a clinical standpoint, I believe that when treating neurotic patients the experience of the emotional trauma (a constant configuration) is present in their unconscious awareness and so is destined to emerge in the course of the analytic work. In complex cases, as in borderline states, difficult infantile experiences compromise personality growth and encourage the construction of pathological structures that obliterate memory of the traumatic experience. In these cases a more complicated path of reconstruction is called for because the link between the psychopathology and the trauma is more deeply concealed and consequently less direct.

The emotional story

The considerations I advance stem from the study of extremely complex and intricate issues that require a huge amount of effort to simplify. The importance we give to emotional trauma in the primary relationship has direct consequences to the way in which we listen to our patients; one of the functions of analytic listening is to distinguish between what was created by the infantile trauma and what results from the psychopathological structures. In fact, the close association between emotional trauma and psychopathological development allows us to intuit the degree of complexity of each patient's therapeutic course.

Even if the emotional trauma has had an impact on the structuring of the personality—causing anxiety or arrests in development, and creating psychopathological structures and objects—parts of the unconscious perceptive functions are still present and operating and the analyst must focus his attention on these.

As mentioned before, in more evolved (neurotic) patients and those capable of representation, the traumas of the primary relationship are also expressed in dreams in which the analyst can appear in place of the traumatic object of the past (Giustino, 2009). Bearing an apparently transferral significance, these dreams describe the nature of the traumatic relationship with the past object extremely well.

An example of an apparently transferral traumatic dream was brought by forty-something-year-old Rita. On returning from holiday she said:

"I dreamt of you, doctor. I came to the session but your wife was with you in your consulting room. I see you passively stretched out on the couch; you were being analysed by your wife. Then you disappear and your wife tells me that she will be my analyst. But after a short time she sends me away and says she doesn't want to have anything to do with my case. I leave upset and perplexed . . ."

Rita says it is a strange dream that she cannot associate to anything. She does not know why she might have dreamt of me like that; I seemed truly disturbed, passive and dependent on my wife. I have a possible explanation in mind for this dream, even if Rita cannot associate. She knows that my wife is an analyst but this is not the right button for unravelling this dream; her childhood story is more useful.

Rita arrived in Italy about ten years ago, two years before beginning analysis. At that time she was depressed, disorientated, and full of anxiety. She had set out from a country in central Europe, leaving her job, and had gone first to France—where she had relatives—before coming to Italy. The first part of her analysis had concluded with her getting married, which she was very happy about. She is now beginning a new period of analysis, after an interval of almost six years from the first, since her marriage has become very problematic.

Rita had a difficult childhood and adolescence. Her family was very poor and only her mother worked; her alcoholic father stayed at home. In the dream, the person represented as the analyst is her childhood alcoholic father. The strong person in the family was her mother (my wife). At a certain point though, her mother had found a new partner and had left her home and daughters to go and live with him. After my interpretation of the past, the patient remembers that she often passed by her mother's and new companion's house and felt she had been totally forgotten. Her mother brought the patient to live with her only later on, once her economic difficulties had been overcome.

The dream plays out a repetition of the infantile trauma down to the smallest details, including being abandoned by her mother (my wife saying she wanted nothing more to do with her). Perhaps we can say that the holiday break from analysis had made Rita lose her relationship with the analyst as a new object enabling the old objects—her parents and all their complications—come to the surface once more.

The emotional trauma in the transference

When the patient is unable to recount his own story, the experience of the primary relationship trauma that he is not aware of often becomes evident in the transference. For example, I had not succeeded in understanding much about a thirty-something-year-old woman called Susanna. In our first encounters she was very tense, almost completely expressionless; perhaps she was trying to understand who I was rather than communicate something of herself.

*   *   *

Susanna's analysis began at two sessions a week due to time constraints and money problems, with the commitment to increase the number as soon as it was possible. We did not mention this again until the patient, after the Easter holiday break, accused me of having forced her to accept three sessions a week starting from a future date. Since I was certain that I had never broached the argument again, I thought she was talking about someone else and not about me. With a stretch of the imagination, I thought she was substituting me for her father, about whom I only had the vaguest information.

From that moment on, part of the analysis was devoted to her relationship with her father, a truly tyrannical figure who had arrogated (and was still claiming) the right to enter into his daughter's life without any consideration for her personality. It had taken a great deal of imagination on my part to intuit how the patient as a child had related to such a parent, what a submissive level she must have reached to be able to live with him, only to distance herself from him later and escape into isolation.

I understood that Susanna had had to restrain her development since she was unable to count on her mother either, also entirely in his thrall. Only later could the analysis tackle some of the patient's specific issues, such as, for example, her angry response to frustration and her tendency to live at a distance from any real human contact. Susanna always seemed to be seeking gratification (in fact she had been entrusted to a grandmother in her early years, for whom she was the privileged object); unable to find any, she slipped easily into the role of victim (as had occurred with me on returning from the Easter break).

Despite the experience with her father being really traumatic, her reaction had been to bind herself masochistically to the traumatic object. She responded aggressively and self-pityingly on a number of occasions in the transference: for example, when I was obliged to ask her to change the time of a session. She reacted violently at that, accusing me of being overbearing and of wanting to traumatise her.

* * *

The pathological response of the primary object is often reproduced from the very first phases in the analytic process and projected on to the figure of the analyst. If the analyst knows how to take the story of the patient's emotional development into himself and give it value, the pathogenic interrelationship with the primary object, which surfaces immediately in analysis, will trigger an appropriate response from him.

I would like to point out that my analytic stance in the case of the patient above was not limited to merely interpreting the transference ("you perceive me as you perceived your father when . . .") but took on a more active role: as well as interpreting the confusion (and projection) between me and her domineering father, I endeavoured to transmit to her my intuitions about her emotional childhood events, before she was capable of doing this for herself.

This approach makes up part of my methodology and I endeavour to use it as soon as possible; I find it helps the patient to distinguish between the *analyst-object of the past* and the *analyst who helps to understand the past*. Interpreting the transference in this case helps to extricate the figure of the analyst as a new potential object from the experience with the internalised objects of the past. Indeed, the analyst's task is to transform the role assigned him by the patient and become a potential new object.

My point of view differs from that of other colleagues (among whom Betty Joseph, 1985) who do not believe it is useful to reconstruct the childhood story until the analysis is far advanced. Joseph's position stems from misgivings that if the past is reconstructed too early, there might be a risk of the patient talking about emotional reality in an intellectualising way rather than experiencing it in the transference relationship with the analyst.

Other post-Kleinian authors, for example, Segal (1991), do not share this idea and do not think that interpretations of the past stray far from those centred on the analysand–analyst relationship. For Rosenfeld (1987), reconstructive interpretations should be considered essential components of the transference and must be given meaning every time they appear. Furthermore, in the case of patients who have suffered trauma, Rosenfeld believes that from the very beginning the analyst should commit himself to a shared clarifying of past events in all their possible effects and concatenations. Indeed, what is striking in many cases is not so much the extraordinary nature of the trauma, but the lack of a human environment capable of sharing, containing, and eventually transforming its impact.

During the analytic process, reconstruction should involve making the patient aware of the memory and reliving it together, because the analyst's emotional participation is an indispensable element for transformation. In these cases the trauma is not projected back into the transference (unless the analyst lends himself to gross distortions), but is relived and transformed in the relationship. The analyst is, therefore, called on to be the object that was lacking in the past traumatic experience.

I, too, believe that the analyst must formulate reconstructive hypotheses at an early stage, even if he can communicate them only when the patient is capable of understanding them. I think that the analyst must evaluate the best moment for doing this, bearing in mind the patient's personality, his ability to understand, and the use he may make of it—all elements that are independent of the length of the analysis and that differ from case to case.

But is it really possible to recover the past in every case?

I think we can answer yes, it is possible, on condition that the patient is equipped with an unconscious capable of emotional thought and associative memory. This function is active to a large extent in neurotic functioning, but very deteriorated, if not absent, in borderline and psychotic patients. In these cases, in the early stages of therapy, we may witness reconstructions of the past that have absolutely no bearing on reality; the truth can emerge only at a more advanced stage when the patient is more capable of emotional insight.

As an example, I asked a young patient of mine, who had come to analysis after a psychotic episode, for some information about his childhood and his parents. He said he had had a happy childhood and he had had a wonderful relationship with his parents; indeed, he could not recall a single instance of being reprimanded or punished. Only later during the analysis, as his capacity for emotional under-standing developed, did it become clear to him that his parents had seemed good because they had been emotionally absent. In fact, the patient had been left alone, completely to his own devices, and had learnt to shut himself away in a fantastic, megalomaniac world, totally neglected by his parents, which subsequently led him towards psychotic development.

Pathological consequences of trauma

In the sphere of the more complex psychic disorders, it is important to differentiate the pathological structures that originated from a precocious intrusion of the primary objects from those that imply active construction on the part of the patient. In some cases, what springs to the fore is not true traumatic suffering, but the absence of any structuring of the mind during infant life.

If the child lives in a world devoid of emotional response on the part of his parents, he cannot develop the representations that are fundamental for creating his sense of reality. Sometimes, the parents' psychic absence fosters pleasurable flight into a world of the imagi-nation to the detriment of contact with psychic reality. This is one of the reasons why a certain number of patients who have, indeed, had a traumatic childhood are quite unaware of this fact. In my opinion, two equally important factors, destined to reinforce each other, concur in encouraging the psychopathology of difficult patients: a lack of empathy from the context around the child, coupled with the child's own constructing of psychopathological structures that will divert him from the path of normal development. The psychopathological structures—specific to each patient—develop precociously and, although connected to the nature of the primary objects and to their interaction with the patient, acquire a stable and autonomous configuration over time.

What trauma?

To demonstrate how psychopathological construction can precede the trauma proper, I will take up my reflections on sexual abuse once again. As mentioned in the previous chapter, a huge amount of analytical literature (especially North American) has reassessed—a century on—Freud's observation on the pathogenic importance of early sexual trauma. All the authors agree in emphasising the pathogenic consequences of the traumatic experience of abuse. Most frequently, it is a father or an adult who abuses a little girl, although this can often be a little boy. The commonest consequences are emotional dissociation, selective scotoma of the event, inhibition of emotional development, frigidity, and so on. But what is not sufficiently highlighted is the importance of the pre-existing conditions of whoever suffered the abuse.

*   *   *

Thirty-two-year-old Marta still looks rather adolescent; of slim build, she is well toned, due to relentlessly practising a number of sports.[4] This frenetic activity—exerting her body in sport and, as will increasingly emerge during analysis, in sexual activities—goes to make up a well structured defence against an underlying depression.

Marta lives alone and undoubtedly escaped a depressed and highly conformist family that did not protect her. A few months after starting analysis, she confesses that when she was twelve, she was regularly molested by her maternal grandfather, who forced her to give him oral sex. Marta never told anyone because she suspected that her sister, and above all her mother, had also been victims of abuse in their turn by grandfather and father.

Immediately after these revelations, having broken the long family code of silence, she questioned her mother and sister, who both confirmed her suspicions. No further reaction followed from the family and everything was once more clothed in silence. However, apart from finding out about the trauma she had suffered, the meaning of sexuality became a sort of guiding thread in Marta's analysis that was ever present from that moment. The sexualisation of relationships and the resulting confusion seem to be a proposal for a cure, as in this dream:

"I'm in a foreign city. I come to meet you, doctor, in a building flooded with water, as though we were in Venice. I meet you in a room and you propose having sex. I'm confused because I don't know whether I want to or not; then I decide that I don't want to and calmly tell you. The thing that puzzled me though was that the water rose and rose and I had to leave, feeling sad. The room was dark; we were talking on a bed. I said to myself: 'I'm usually up for all kinds of experiences; I had even imagined this one as being possible but now I no longer desire it.'"

In this first dream, for Marta a *sexual cure* is more or less the same thing as a proposal for therapy; analytic intimacy can be transformed in the sexualised confusion of infancy. The house of the dream is not an appropriate place in which to welcome her (it does not hold water) and the analyst—cold and distant—plays the role of an adult person dominated by incestuous desire.

After the first year of analysis, the patient progressively distanced herself from this sexualised mental state and in her life, too, the compulsive episodes and sexual promiscuity diminished. In her dreams, compulsive sex no longer appears as an arousing and beneficial cure but, on the contrary, seems to threaten the good emotional experiences. In fact, in this period, attraction for sexualised confusion was often symbolised as a dangerous occurrence that triggers anxiety.

So, what connection is there, then, between the sexualised arousal that invaded Marta's early life and that conditions her adult life and the childhood trauma? Her sexuality was not inhibited by her grandfather's abuse; on the contrary, it seems to have acquired its own life over the years, independent from the sexual trauma: did the abuse activate the sexualisation of Marta's mind or was the trauma grafted on to a process of sexualisation that preceded it?

* * *

In a session towards the end of the second year of her analysis, Marta dreams that

> "an aunt places a piece of furniture in such a way that it prevents access to the room in which the sexual encounters with the grandfather took place". She remembers that she used to hide alone in masturbatory withdrawal behind that same sofa: "I don't know if it was in the dream or in my child-hood [referring to the sofa or the sitting room] I used to hide behind this sofa and it had something to do with my sexuality, but I was alone . . ."

If we use this dream to reconstruct childhood events, we have to infer that the state of masturbatory sexual arousal must have preceded the sexual abuse. We can conjecture that the sexual trauma was inscribed within an earlier sexualised withdrawal, probably created in answer to a lack of affective maternal communication. For this reason, the trauma, instead of inhibiting sexuality, permitted the primitive sexualisation—born as an excited defence—to accompany the patient throughout her life and development.

Trauma and self-pitying withdrawal

While some patients have no recollection of infantile emotional trau-mas, which generally emerge only later on during analysis, others communicate them right from the very beginning. They accurately describe their parents' characters, what they lacked, and the injustices they suffered; it seems as though they record every wrong done to them, whether inevitable or fortuitous, so they can excite themselves in a mental refuge full of resentment and violence. The analyst's emotional participation does not bring them any relief; in fact, it seems to intensify the gravity of their grievances. Denouncing past suffering reinforces their position of victim and fuels an increasing aggressiveness.

*   *   *

The analysis of a young woman, named Carmen, is dominated by endless accusations against her parents, especially her mother, whose emotional distance triggers uncontainable rages. But Carmen is tied to her mother in a double bind: at the same time, she is also in a position of psychological submission and total dependence. In the course of her life, she meets people who turn out to be tyrannical and violent; she tried to have a sentimental relationship with someone but it soon developed into a perverse relationship in which she, apparently passively, was subjected to both physical and sexual abuse.

Carmen's relationship with her mother represents the main source of her sadomasochistic storms. Recently, she had to take a train to go to another town and had asked her mother for money so that she could get a taxi to return home from the station as she would have arrived late at night. When her mother refused, she had not made any objection, appearing to accept that decision. However, as soon as she got off the train, she felt herself engulfed by violence: "When I got off the train I didn't have any money for a taxi and I no longer remembered where the bus stop was. I went out into the square in front of the station and it was dark. I saw a group of drunk African guys who were throwing bottles of beer around. The fact is that I wasn't afraid of that gang at all . . . I could have avoided them, I could have gone a different way, but instead I went right through them . . . as if to say . . . it's already happened to me once, what's going to be so bad about a second time? That's what I do when I cut myself; it's like in the concentration camps, you become an object without emotions."

*   *   *

On this occasion, the patient is more interested in demonstrating how awful the world is (men and her mother) than in protecting herself; she finds greater pleasure in provoking the aggression than in defending herself. Offering herself as a victim of rape testifies to her relentless masochistic rage and the role she plays of aggressive victim.

Steiner (1993) postulates that specific pathological organisations are at the basis of these states of *resentment* and *revenge*, which can be understood as passive, masochistic, or manic defences against feelings of guilt that the patient is unable to accept. Chronically feeling oneself to be the victim of wrong serves to avoid questioning one's own share of responsibility and implies not working through the mourning for the trauma suffered and for what has been lost in the past that is no longer recoverable. Traumatic suffering is transformed into a chronic struggle in which the object is tortured but the relationship with it is never broken; the perverse satisfaction obtained through arousal in the counter-aggressive circle makes change increasingly difficult.

The therapeutic relationship

It is difficult to understand what really contributes to analytic trans-formation and to repairing the traumatic experience. Where does change begin? How can a relationship be formed that is capable of producing a new development in patients that are difficult to cure?

In the past, the heart of analytic work lay in interpreting the trans-ference. This way of seeing things originated with Freud's views on neurosis, on the repressed infantile conflict, and on its reproduction in the transference. Freud believed it was necessary to interpret the transference in order to gain access to the memory and to nurture awareness.

However, in the treatment of difficult patients, it is necessary to trust above all in the analytic relationship because it can develop a new bond of dependence whose purpose is mental growth. In fact, a large part of the therapeutic process depends on the capacity of the two players—analyst and analysand—to create *a relationship that aids development*. For this reason, I distinguish the transference and the countertransference from the analytic relationship.

More simply, we can say that while the *transference* is prevalently the work of the patient's projections, and of his split *parts* and child-hood past, the *analytic relationship* is a new construction that results from the meeting of the analysand's and the analyst's receptive parts, and that develops with help from both of them.

In particular, the analytic relationship depends on the analyst's skill in creating and maintaining in his mind *a place* (Di Chiara, 1985) for the patient, considered as an individual with his own story, his emotional difficulties, and his implicit request for mental growth, and on the patient's willingness to consider the analyst as a *transformational object* (Bollas, 1979); in other words, as an object that is necessary for development. As long as this basic bond remains alive, the analytic process continues and advances.

As already mentioned, the transference, the countertransference, and the analytic relationship are processes that coexist and recipro-cally influence each other. Indeed, the transference is not based only on the patient's projections and on his past, but also on the analyst's conscious and unconscious responses. For example, a negative trans-ference, which might recall the way in which the patient reacted to his father in infancy, can be aided by an unempathetic attitude on the part of the analyst. Let us remember, at this point, that Freud's concept of *unobjectivable transference* was the first attempt to theorise the realm of the analytic relationship and mental growth.

In other words, the analytic relationship is based on a natural need to depend on an object for mental growth and the nature of this relationship depends on the analyst's receptivity and on the quality of his emotional response to the patient's communications. The analytic relationship is directed towards the future and, for difficult patients, is the space in which new emotional experiences that have never been experienced before take shape. These unknown experiences require participation and sharing. The concrete reality of the traumatic experience impeded the development of the patient's potential space; this obstacle is destined to last until a new object and a new experience, sometimes never experienced before, will begin to be present in the patient's inner world. I speak about this aspect of the analytic relationship in Chapter Nine, on discussing the loving transference, when the feelings of love for the analyst represent a new affective experience that was obstructed in the past. In this case, when appropriately treated, the infantile loving transference starts the patient off towards an adult emotional relationship.

In these two chapters, I have attempted to define a series of concatenations between the traumatic experience, in particular the precocious one, the memory of it, and its effects on the maturing individual. As can be seen, the interlacing of it all is highly complex.

One point of view that is very present in contemporary literature tends to consider all experiences that disturb the development of infant emotivity to be traumatic, especially the relationships in which the mother does not provide empathetic responses to her child's requests for emotional contact and does not answer to his need for containment and personality structuring.

Frustration can be included among empathetic responses because it serves to structure the mind; it should, by no means, always be considered traumatic. A mother has to know how to distinguish between her child's needs and his claims for domination. A correct dose of frustration serves to contain a child's demands for omnipotence and attribute substance to the personality of whoever is on the receiving end.

CHAPTER FOUR

Defences and psychopathological constructions

"If the love object responds indifferently to love, the heart is replaced by an empty hole, not just a passive void, a bottle with no bottom, but a place that actively drains all substance and evacuates the good together with the bad in vengeful resentment"

(Anzieu & Monjauze, 2004, p. 41)

In this chapter, I attempt to illustrate a characteristic feature of difficult patients that makes their analysis particularly complex and arduous. I do this by differentiating the defences from psychopathological constructions, which are characteristic of complex pathologies such as borderline states, sexual perversions, and psychotic states. I devote the first part of the chapter to looking at how the concept of defence is treated first in the Freudian model (defence against instinct) and then in the Kleinian model (defence against anxiety), and after that go on to discuss the psychopathological construction, which assumes a pathogenic power that the patient is quite unaware of. The notion of the psychopathological construction or structure, advanced by post-Kleinian authors who have studied the more complex pathologies, has not, unfortunately, received the attention it merits from contemporary psychoanalytic practice.

However, in order to differentiate the defences from psychopathological constructions, we must begin by briefly describing the different ways of theorising the defences that underlie the two models—the instinctual one and the object-relations one.

Sigmund Freud

In "The neuro-psychoses of defence" (1894a), Freud describes three forms of hysteria: the first, *retention hysteria*, represents a morbid state in which an affect has not been adequately abreacted; the second, *hypnoid hysteria*, is characterised by a mental—in fact, hypnoid—state in which mental representations are not integrated but remain dissociated; the third, *defence hysteria*, is characterised by defensive activity against representations that cause unpleasant affects. Within this last form of hysteria, Freud formulates the notion of defence for the first time, and it will remain fundamental throughout the development of psychoanalytic theory.

In the subsequent *Studies on Hysteria* (Freud, 1895d) the distinction between the three forms of hysteria is still maintained, although defence hysteria gains in importance at the expense of the hypnoid state, whose action in generating hysteria was upheld by Breuer. After breaking with Breuer, Freud concentrated almost exclusively on defence hysteria, dropping the term *defence* in subsequent works, in which he refers only to hysteria.

This focus on *defence* represented a turning point in psychoanalysis and led to the formulation of a cardinal concept that would have specific implications for the genesis of mental illness. From that moment, defence, with its corresponding concept of conflict, would, in the psychoanalytic sphere, characterise the entire realm of psychopathology, derived from the study of defence hysteria proposed earlier and then dismissed.

Why was the specific term *defence* discarded? For the simple reason that, from then on, Freud maintained that defensive activity occurred in every manifestation of mental life. Consequently, if every psychopathology was the result of conflict and defence, why highlight it only for hysteria?

Defence has a compulsive nature; it works in an unconscious way and is directed against impulses that might provoke unpleasant effects for the ego. In *New Introductory Lectures on Psycho-analysis*, Freud (1933a) mentions only four defences as being truly important: repression, sublimation, displacement, and reaction formation.

In "Some psychical consequences of the anatomical distinction between the sexes" Freud (1925j) describes disavowal as a process, present in children of both sexes, directed towards denying the absence of a penis in the female. In contrast to repression, this defence can be the point of departure for psychosis in an adult: while the neurotic represses the demands of the id (instinct), the psychotic disavows reality.

With "Fetishism", Freud (1927e) begins to develop the notion of denial with particular reference to fetishism, in which two incompatible positions coexist: the perception of female castration and its disavowal.

In subsequent works ("Splitting of the ego in the process of defence", 1940e; *An Outline of Psycho-Analysis*, 1940a), the notion of ego splitting accompanies that of disavowal. The two attitudes of the fetishist, who oscillates between denying the lack of a penis in the woman and being gripped by anxiety on recognising this, persist alongside each other without ever meeting precisely because of the split in the ego.

Anna Freud

The task of methodically organising the defences was tackled by Anna Freud (1961) in *The Ego and the Mechanisms of Defence*.

> There are an extraordinarily large number of methods (or mechanisms, as we say) used by our ego in the discharge of its defensive functions. An investigation is at this moment being carried on close at hand which is devoted to the study of these methods of defence: my daughter, the child analyst, is writing a book upon them. (Freud, 1936a, p. 244)

Anna Freud postulates that the defences operate in a very wide-ranging field; as well as being directed against danger from within, they also serve to evade danger from the outside world. In some cases, by denying the existence of the real sources of fear or pain, the defence limits the function of the ego because it upsets the ego's powers for critically examining reality and recognising objects.

According to Anna Freud, the defences are not only pathological mechanisms, but also appear during age-linked changes. In adolescence, for example, intellectualising and a certain tendency towards asceticism serve to distance the individual from instinctual impulses that are preparing to burst into his life.

This chapter does not aim to pursue in greater detail the development of these ideas by important trends in current, especially North American, analytic thought (for more on this, see Lingiardi & Madeddu, 2002). I would merely like to point out that ego psychology (Heinz Hartmann, Ernst Kris, and Rudolph Lowenstein) took up Anna Freud's idea that defensive measures of a physiological type gradually become real defence mechanisms. This group conceptualised defences as adaptive functions that the ego can make use of to integrate instinctual demands with those of external reality.

Melanie Klein

Klein introduced a radical departure in the way the defences are theorised. For her, the defences are unavoidable stages of mental growth that aim to set the immature ego off on the path towards development; the primitive defences guarantee that the little integrated ego will, in fact, mature. Many of the cases described in *The Psycho-Analysis of Children* (Klein, 1950) adhere to this model.

Whereas in Freud's view the *defences originate from the instinctual conflict,* in Klein's view they serve to modulate or to *project excessive anxiety outside the individual and so protect the ego.* The paranoid–schizoid and the depressive positions are, at the same time, defences against anxiety and specific ways of relating to the object. Defences can be equated to primitive mechanisms because they serve the immature ego; they become pathological when they are no longer useful for development.

It is generally said that the defences described by Melanie Klein are psychotic defences as opposed to those described by Freud, which would be neurotic defences. However, we must make it clear that Klein talks of defence mechanisms of a psychotic type, and not of illness or of the psychotic state. Psychotic defences are precocious defences that the individual uses in the primitive phase, the paranoid–schizoid stage of his development; they are of a psychotic type *because they are precocious* and not *vice versa*.

Projective identification

The specific defence mechanism of the psychotic states identified by Klein is *projective identification* (1946), described in "Notes on some schizoid mechanisms". As formulated, projective identification implies projecting parts of the subject's self into an object. In this way, the person projecting perceives himself as identified with the object, which finds itself containing parts of the projected self, or even feeling controlled by the object in whom the projection happened.

An exhaustive description of projective identification can be found in the essay "On identification" (Klein, 1955), which takes its cue from Julien Green's novel, *If I Were You* (1950). The protagonist, Fabien, a man in crisis and depressed, enters the body of a person he envies, taking on this person's qualities. But, after repeating this experience a number of times, each time becoming the person he has taken possession of, he becomes increasingly impoverished and ends by feeling claustrophobic. At the end, Fabien has to carry out a complex operation to regain possession of his original identity.

Klein tells us that the subject's ego becomes impoverished due to the effects of projective identification because it confuses itself with the object of the projection: for this reason, she believes that this operation is a defence (for example, against envy) and not a communication.

Starting with Bion, who described a projective identification used with a communicative aim, this concept was given a much wider significance by post-Kleinian analysts compared to its original meaning. Projective identification used with a communicative aim would be a primitive form of object relations, or, in other words, a *communicative projection*. The expanded meaning assigned to this mechanism in post-Kleinian literature went hand in hand with the increasing importance attributed to the countertransference in analytical practice.

Even though Kleinian analysts sustain that projective identification becomes pathological when it is used excessively, we can say that the difference between communicative projection and projective identification does not depend only on the intensity, but above all on what is projected.

In normal projective identification (or communicative projection), a feeling is projected with the hope that it is welcomed and understood by the object (the baby cries desperately and the mother intuitively responds). In pathological projective identification, on the other hand, parts of the self—usually undesired ones—are projected and the desired parts are appropriated; this impoverishes the self and leads to a state of confusion between what belongs to the subject and what to the object.

I believe we can use the term *communicative projection* to refer to the mechanism of normal projective identification rather than to the pathological process described by Klein for psychotic patients. As she states, when parts of the self are projected, the result is confusion between self and object, something that does not occur in communicative projection.

Post-Kleinian thought

Eric Brenman, an author from the Kleinian group, has, in my view, reflected very creatively on the dual aspect of defence. Returning to a statement by Freud (1937c) in which he postulates that defences serve to hold danger at bay but can also, in their turn, be transformed into danger, the British analyst advances an analogy between defence and skin, made up of dead cells. The protective layer of the epidermis, in other words its defence, cannot be too thin because it would lose its protective function, but neither can it be too thick, as it would then risk suffocating the organism that can no longer communicate with the outside world. Excessive defence produces mental deficiency.

Brenman writes, "All defences create a delusion or illusion and cannot operate without corruption and mutilation of the perceptual apparatus" (2006, p. 39). In the author's opinion, from the very beginning of life, awareness of external and internal reality (our feelings, passions, and fears) is unbearable unless there is someone who understands our needs and helps us tolerate the intensity of our feelings: the more we are able to accept this help, the less we are obliged to have recourse to defences. Even if they can save us from catastrophe, psychic defences, in any case, distort our capacity to cope with the truth and limit our openness towards others.

According to Brenman, in the early phases of life truth can be distorted in order to survive, but it is gradually recognised as the depressive position advances. He emphasises that, once established, the primitive defence mechanisms tend to prevail over the more evolved mechanisms acquired subsequently. This explains why, in moments of crisis, the primitive defences once again take the upper hand and regression is easy. The traumatic experience, too, tends to trigger the same primitive defences; in general, the defences are nurtured by primitive parts. On the occasion of the presentation of his book in Milan (Brenman, 2002), I asked Brenman if the trauma creates psychopathological structures and if these differ from defences; he responded that the trauma develops the primitive parts and that defences are fuelled by primitive parts. In short, Brenman, in line with other post-Kleinian authors, does not believe in the existence of pathological defences that are different from the omnipotent defences brought into action by the primitive ego.

Psychopathological constructions

The hypothesis I put forward is that in the more complex pathologies it is not sufficient to talk merely of primitive defences, which certainly exist, we must also consider the action of the *psychopathological constructions*. A psychopathological construction is something more than, and different from, a primitive defence: it represents a new construction that is not present during primary development. Psychopathological constructions are formed silently in infancy and only subsequently express their pathogenic potential; often stimulated by emotional traumas, they soon develop independently.

My point of view is that the psychopathological nuclei that sustain the state of illness in more complex patients do not correspond to the primitive mechanisms present in the early phases of development. *Pathological is not a synonym for primitive.*

This brings me to differ from post-Kleinian authors for whom the psychopathology is fuelled by defences that can be useful and physiological in early infancy, but which become pathogenic if they persist in following stages. Instead, I believe that in subjects destined to fall ill, specific structures are formed right from infancy that are not found in normal development. While they are primitive, psychopathological constructions do not correspond to normal infantile defences; they grow together with the personality that is maturing and remain latent until expressing their pathogenic potential later.

The distinction between defences and *psychopathological constructions* or *organisations* provides us with a better viewpoint when treating difficult cases, where mental structures that cannot be defined as defences come into play. When defences such as repression or projection are used, the unconscious perception of the defensive transformation under way is preserved, while, in the presence of a psychopathological construction, a radical alteration in awareness and personality structure occurs.

Psychotic operating

In short, we can say that psychopathological constructions tend to bring the subject into the realm of psychosis, whereas the defences operate in the sphere of the neuroses.

Unlike the defences, which do not completely destroy awareness, the psychopathological constructions tend to distort psychic reality until it is destroyed: the pathological reality is presented as being superior and more desirable and seduces the patient. Getting rid of such mental states is extremely difficult and leaves behind a state of deep anxiety and depersonalisation precisely because emotional perception has been so completely destroyed. This type of construction is evident in the perversions, and in borderline and psychotic states in which the patient can regress hypnotically towards a state of pleasurable withdrawal that removes him from emotional reality.

I believe that if we adhere to the concept of defence as a primitive mechanism (Klein) or as an action of adaptation (Anna Freud and the ego psychologists), we cannot completely understand the psychopathological reality of the more complex mental conditions.

The fact that the word "defence" cannot encompass a number of important aspects of clinical reality is also confirmed by assertions advanced by a number of authors from the Kleinian group. Even though these remain bound to the paranoid–schizoid and depressive positions, O'Shaughnessy (1981), for example, distinguishes the defence from the *defensive organisation*. She writes.

> Unlike defences—piecemeal, transient to a greater or lesser extent, recurrent—which are a normal part of development, a defensive organisation is a fixation, a pathological formation when development arouses irresoluble and almost overwhelming anxiety. Expressed in Kleinian terms, defences are a normal part of negotiating the paranoid–schizoid and depressive positions; a defensive organisation, on the other hand, is a pathological fixed formation in one or other position, or on the borderline between them. (1981, p. 362)

In particular, psychopathological constructions are triggered by infantile traumatic experiences. This origin is not explicitly recognised by those post-Kleinian authors who identified the importance and function of the pathological organisations. Rosenfeld (1964), for example, sustains that the *constellation of interrelated defences*, typical of narcissistic patients, serves specifically to distance them from the pain connected to object dependence or to defend them from envy.

In contrast, I believe that the psychopathological construction originates from a failed relationship or from a lack of objects useful for development: if the child does not find nourishment outside, he will turn inwards and to his fantastic world, which, in this way, ends by replacing the relational world. In other words, the pain to defend oneself against originates from experiences of traumatic infantile relationships and not from a hatred of dependence. In this sense, it is more useful to understand the way in which the patient was obliged to construct and use the psychopathological construction than to highlight its anti-relational nature.

Destructive narcissism

Some authors (Spillius, 1983; Steiner, 1982) have proposed the term *pathological organisation* to highlight how the pathological structure can become part of the self.

The author who clarified the operational modes of the psychopathological structure was Herbert Rosenfeld (1971) with his description of destructive narcissism. He hypothesises that in some serious psychopathologies, an internal bad agent is idealised, a bad self, that corresponds to a psychotic part that distances the person from contact with his emotions and from relationships with others. The sick parts are idealised and wield power over the rest of the self; in particular, the destructive and self-destructive part would intimidate or seduce those parts of the person more capable of insight, attracting and ensnaring them. The concept of destructive narcissism cannot be generalised, but must be used in specific contexts. It is a psycho-pathological construction that concerns borderline and perverse patients and also some psychotics. It implies a psychic withdrawal to a secret area in which the patient is imprisoned in a highly patholog-ical system.

The psychopathological structure is similar to a delusional object that successfully persuades the subject's healthy parts to be ensnared because they can then delude themselves they are quite free of pain and free to indulge in every transgressive activity. The same goes for sadomasochistic perversion, in which the pleasure of transgressing—"you can do absolutely anything you want"—lies at the basis of sexual ecstasy (De Masi, 2003[1999]).

The destructive narcissism of these patients is organised in the same way as a gang of delinquents dominated by a leader who controls all its members with the sole aim of intensifying their destruc-tive activity.

The main problem with this type of patients is that they perpetu-ally live in a state of inner confusion between what is good and constructive and what is destructive, and the confusion has to be constantly analysed. A pathological superego aligned with the sick part of the self often exists; for this reason, obedience must be blind and any insubordination is punished by threatening attacks and accu-sations. When this type of patient improves, he often dreams of being attacked by members of the Mafia or by groups of delinquent adoles-cents.

The psychopathological construction cannot be considered a simple expression of the mechanisms of primitive idealisation, but represents a pathological distortion of psychic development, or, in other words, an idealisation of a bad part of the self. Its supremacy is the result of the perverse transformation of the superego that makes it seem as though destructiveness is innocent and exciting.

* * *

Only after two years of analysis and after a trusting relationship had been established with the analyst could Vittorio, a young disturbed patient, a drug addict and suicidal, allow any exploration of the destructive withdrawal within which he had been imprisoned for a long time. This refuge is inhabited by Nero, a tyrannical character with whom Vittorio has identified because he represents uncontrolled destructiveness. Whenever he is opposed, Vittorio–Nero flies into a rage and, putting himself in the place of a wrongly persecuted victim, legitimates his right for revenge. So, as Nero destroys, sacks, and sets fire to the city, he feels perverse pleasure in spreading confusion and violence among his love objects.

* * *

The power the pathological organisation acquires over the rest of the self depends on the role of the superego, which is perverse and unlike its primitive counterpart described by Klein. Indeed, while in some clinical situations we find ourselves in front of a superego in which the primitive aspects are well to the fore, in the case of the psychopathological structures an intimidating superego with a perverse nature is at work (see Chapter Six).

Brenman (2002) describes a cruel superego that dominates the self; to maintain the idealisation of the cruel aspects requires a considerable restriction of perception and an attendant mental paucity.

The delinquent gang

I wanted to emphasise the difference between defence and psychopathological organisation to show that we are in front of two structures that differ in meaning and outcome, even though they both spring from a defensive need. Pathological organisation is similar to delusion, aiming to subjugate the emotional and relational part of the patient, which acts against the vital parts of the self. It emerges as a split structure that can assume different aspects such as, for example, the figure of a splendid character who promises the patient a state of well-being. This world seems very pleasurable and seductive as long as the patient submits to it, but takes on a threatening nature when he attempts to evade it. The equilibrium is always very unstable and, in any case, tipped in favour of the psychopathological part. Our analytic work lies above all in constantly clarifying for the patient the meaning of the psychopathological organisation and the means it uses to enthral him.

* * *

Twenty-three-year-old Gabriele had given up his studies and no longer left his house, immersed in a world of gratifying fantasies, like a second Oblomov. After years of analytic work and just as he was beginning to have a bit more contact with reality, he described in a dream his attempt to free himself from the pathological organisation that held him hostage:

> "I was at a party, there were a lot of people and I had a gun in my hand; I was part of a gang of delinquents who kidnapped people . . . the aim was to attack and rob them . . . then I shot two of the gang from behind. I woke up full of anxiety."

* * *

It is obvious that his anxiety is linked to the threat of retaliation wielded over him by the psychotic organisation in the moment he tries to escape its clutches. This dream is pretty typical: the psychopathological organisation is often represented as a gang of delinquents (Meltzer, 1973; Rosenfeld, 1971) as a way of underlining its power and perverse objective. In the dream, it is significant that Gabriele at first appears as part of the gang (he complies with its power) but then attempts to defy it.

At times the gang represents a pathological superego, as in the following clinical vignette.

* * *

A doctor of about forty, who came to analysis for a depressive state that has accompanied him since early childhood, arrives for the session in a state of great anxiety. One of his relatives has just been diagnosed with a serious illness. A few months previously, the doctor had by chance seen some of this person's routine medical test results—requested by the GP—which were all normal. He feels he is to blame for not having looked into the matter further, and relates this dream:

> he is with a friend in the very squalid suburbs of the city, and sees a group of drug addicts, two of whom come towards him. He knows he must not

avert his eyes as the addicts, who look like real delinquents, would then approach in a much more threatening way. At a certain point he sees a lift and walks towards it to go up. As he is getting into it, one of the addicts comes up to him and tries to take some money—a modest sum—from his pocket. His friend urges him to give the money to the addict but he resists because he knows that if he does not oppose him this delinquent will rob him of everything.

*   *   *

The superego here seems to have assumed the form of a delinquent organisation that threatens to dominate the patient completely. For this reason, in his dream he tries to defy it. In everyday life, this doctor, who has suffered depressive episodes of clinical severity, seems to be dominated by a constant sense of persecutory guilt that makes him compulsively assist others while completely neglecting his own needs.

CHAPTER FIVE

Psychic withdrawal

"Gradually she became one of the many who do not feel that they exist in their own right as whole human beings. . . . while she was at school and later at work, there was another life going on in terms of the part that was dissociated. [The main part of her] was living in what became an organized sequence of fantasying"

(Winnicott, 1971, p. 29)

P sychic withdrawal is the commonest pathological organisation and the one most fraught with consequences. Conceptualising this mental state allows us to distinguish the transitional area— of play and daydreaming—from the area that impedes psychic and emotional development and confines the child to a claustrophiliac space. A number of examples illustrate the different types of withdrawal: sensory, identifying with imaginary characters, sexualised, and destructive. In some cases, the infantile withdrawal will become the crucible that gives rise to later psychotic development.

In the preceding chapter, I described the psychopathological constructions of more complex patients, differentiating them from defences that are present in less serious cases.

I would now like to discuss another pathological structure that, in my view, is specific to difficult patients and that is very dangerous because it tends to progressively colonise the healthy part of the self. Steiner's book *Psychic Retreats* (1993) is a very effective and praise-worthy attempt to theorise this form of pathological organisation.

Steiner conceives the psychic retreat as a collection of defence mechanisms and object-relation systems that culminate in establishing a true psychic place to which the subject can withdraw in the presence of emotions that are, for him, unbearable. He writes,

> The retreat then serves as an area of the mind where reality does not have to be faced, where fantasy and omnipotence can exist unchecked and where anything is permitted. This feature is often what makes the retreat so attractive to the patient and commonly involves the use of perverse or psychotic mechanisms. (Steiner, 1993, p. 3)

Operating to protect the patient from paranoid–schizoid and depressive anxiety, the retreat can take on a variety of aspects that range from full immersion in a romantic fairy-tale world in which everything is idealised, up to masturbatory withdrawal under the dictates of pornographic excitation. These retreats are ruled by omnipotent fantasy, perverse relations, sadomasochism, and narcissism, all elements that provide the self with a sensation of pseudo-self-confidence and pseudo-protection.

The chief consequences of activating pathological organisations, according to Steiner, are withdrawal from object relations and inhibition of the processes of psychic development. In analysis, the existence of a retreat is signalled by the appearance in dreams of violent perverse addictive structures (sects, totalitarian regimes, delinquent or Mafia gangs), or of abandoned houses, grottoes, fortresses, or islands to which the subject withdraws.

The withdrawal, as I prefer to call it, can persist over a long time but is not destined to remain static; indeed, it usually expands and takes over the rest of the self. This explains the pathogenic power of some retreats that, after being established in childhood, can lead to a psychotic episode in adulthood. Parents who are psychologically absent often do not notice that their child is not the gentle, calm person he seems to be, but has, in fact, already withdrawn into a world apart where he is constructing his psychopathology. Since withdrawing progressively alters contact with emotional reality and erases any perception of being abandoned or of the parent's emotional absence, these children do not signal their discomfort. To avoid difficult or traumatic emotional experiences, such as an absent or perpetually anxious and intrusive mother, some of them will construct a retreat. In these cases, interference of an environmental nature results in them failing to experience good dependence. It is important to remember that, once set in motion, the process advances autonomously.

Withdrawal is a defensive measure but also, and above all, a pleasurable place in which the patient feels capable of creating his own objects from nothing. This place must be kept secret at all costs to safeguard its continuing existence, and this is exactly what happens in the analysis of these patients, who only communicate the presence of this secret place at an advanced stage of therapy. Dogged silences in the course of treatment often correspond to moments in which the patient is cultivating the secret space of his withdrawal.

Making use of repeated identifications with fantasy characters, withdrawal has a predominantly sensory nature. This type of pathological structure creates dependence and drains the rest of emotional life, damaging the development of personal identity, at times irreversibly. As mentioned above, psychic withdrawal manifests a variety of configurations, but its overriding characteristic is that of presenting itself as an "other reality" in which the patient lives.

In an earlier work (De Masi, 2006), I distinguished the intuitive imagination from escape into fantasy and emphasised the importance of differentiating positive imaginings—necessary for keeping lines to the future open—from constructions of parallel worlds dissociated from reality. These constructions represent highly pathogenic defences because, even when they do not produce clamorous results, they alter the perceptive–emotional functions necessary for the integration of psychic life. Many of the chapters in the second part of this book are devoted to patients who use psychic withdrawal as an alternative to experiences that serve to maintain contact with reality and mental growth.

I include an example of this when describing the psychic withdrawals that are structured in pathological dependences on the Internet (Chapter Fourteen). Withdrawal into the web world often begins in childhood and starts with an excessive dependence on video games.

* * *

Six-year-old Alberto was brought to a consultation by his mother, worried by his excessive dependence on video games. His fascination with this world does not finish even when he stops playing, but continues for hours. Alberto identifies with the characters of the video game or else invents others. At times, says his mother, he falls to the ground and plays at "being dead". In that moment, he really does not seem part of this world and derives enormous pleasure from this mental state. This so enthralls him, he repeats it again and again. Once, taking advantage of his parents being busy with friends in the garden, he had really disappeared. The grown ups looked for him everywhere and were so worried they alerted the police. Then Alberto suddenly reappeared without a care in the world; indeed, he was amazed at how worried his parents were. He had not given a thought to their preoccupation but hugely enjoyed the idea that he had quite disappeared from their sight, whereas he could see them.

*   *   *

For Alberto, withdrawal into video games and a fantasy world really does seem to be more important than maintaining a bond with reality. His attempts at "being dead" or disappearing for prolonged periods from his parents' sight become an exciting exercise in withdrawing from the world. I have three other cases in mind of adult patients who remember how "disappearing", which for them meant "ending up in another world", had been just as exciting for them when they were little.

The use of the perceptive organs to create artificial states of well-being is what chiefly characterises these states, rather than projection towards the world or curiosity. The fantasised construction of virtual and parallel worlds wields a highly seductive power that prevents the patient from recognising its pathogenic nature.

When these worlds appear in clinical material or in dreams, it is important to describe them in detail to the patient, who substitutes what is pleasurable for what is good and useful for the mind.

Examples of withdrawal types

I shall now briefly mention some psychic withdrawals and trace their development.

Sensory withdrawal

After coming out of a period in hospital, a patient fought her states of desperate solitude by immersing herself in psychotic fantasies: with a lit cigarette in her hand she used to create an ecstatic vision of pleasure, the illusion of being a sheik surrounded by dancing girls. Whenever she came out of this mental state, she was depersonalised and gripped by panic; she could remember nothing about herself or the world she had erased. She then spoke of psychic infarcts.

*   *   *

This example shows how the creation of an "other" sensory reality involves concretely obliterating psychic reality. The patient becomes aware of this only afterwards when the drugged state wears off.

*   *   *

Another example is provided by a twenty-five-year-old patient who came to analysis for a number of reasons, the most important of which, according to him, was a fetish for hair that he had long cherished. This mania had begun when he was little, when he liked to draw girls with long hair; even now he enjoys drying his girlfriend's hair and combing it out. He dreams of having long hair himself and fantasises a long plait swinging behind him. Focusing his fantasies on hair, he reaches an ecstatic state of beatitude, sometimes accompanied by masturbation. This passion for female hair seems to be linked to an infantile eroticised relationship with the body of his mother, whose underclothes he used to wear.

The patient seems very childlike and often speaks in an affected or rather soppy way. In one session, he describes how he had begun to fantasise about hair as soon as he woke up and this had led to wanting to masturbate. But then he had started remembering his schoolfriends of the past and had understood something important about some clashes that had spoiled the relationship with them. "I had felt like masturbating, but after this flash of memories I didn't want to any more. I sensed that these intuitions erased the fantasies that I was having about having long hair."

*   *   *

This is a very important passage. The patient himself begins to differentiate the state of sensory well-being, created by him in the moment he possesses the fetishist object, from the mental state free from the seduction of pleasure, in which he is capable of thinking and reflecting. In this session, the patient seems to demonstrate an initial awareness of the nature of the sensory withdrawal and how it obliterates his capacity to think.

Living as imaginary characters

A father telephones to request an appointment for his daughter[5] who is very unwell: she has not managed to go to school for two years and just stays at home all day. She interrupted psychotherapy two years ago. She sleeps from morning to late afternoon and stays awake at night to communicate with people met on the Internet. Very early in the morning, before dawn, she goes out alone, returning about eight o'clock when the streets are beginning to fill with people on their way to work. Sometimes she stays out, hiding in some dark corner of the city she lives in and her parents have to go and find her and take her back home.

Aged eighteen, Agnese arrives at the first session with her father. She is wearing a long black dress with a sort of nineteenth-century-style cap and at first sight looks as though she might be a nun. Her lips, painted black like her dress, stand out sharply against the deathly pallor of her face.

The conversation comes round to her clothes. Agnese says her dress is dark Gothic Lolita. She does not like it very much because it was made in Italy; she is waiting for some Japanese clothes ordered on the rock singer Mana's website. Mana is a male transvestite; for Agnese he is a god. When she gets the clothes she has ordered, she will become one of Mana's little dolls and feel she belongs to his ranks of special people.

One of the reasons she does not go out during the day is because the sun might make her skin go a different colour from Mana's starchy whiteness.

In subsequent meetings, she describes how she is attracted to the deathly pallor of corpses. She downloads Japanese films from the Internet featuring outrageous characters that fascinate her: cannibalistic situations, stories of prostitutes who have become super-rich, incestuous daughters who murder their father. She is also morbidly attracted to blood; for example, if there is a car accident, she wants to see the injured or dying person.

During clashes with her mother, who does not understand her and who would like to stay glued to her side forever, she repeats destructive fantasies. She wants to be like the star of a series of Japanese cartoons, who can destroy everything she wants with her mind. She, too, hates her mother, who threw her down a well. Agnese believes that witches really exist and have powers conferred on them by demons so they can spread evil everywhere. When she can, she writes short stories or poems, all very desperate, dark, or macabre. She says she hates the world and feels nothing for human suffering. She often fantasises about killing herself because then she could join a school friend she was fond of and who died very young of leukaemia. She barely knew him and adds that two people know each other better if they do not see each other ... She is always watching films with a bloody storyline. She excites herself in this way; she takes part in the evil but knows she is not harming anyone. For some time now she has liked to make small cuts on her arms: she enjoys feeling pain.

Often she cannot sleep, tormented by the vision of two red eyes staring at her. When she has a bath, she is terrified that sooner or later blood will gush out of the taps. Yet, she likes to think of herself as dead, in a state of calm and free of anxiety.

In these sessions, Agnese relates a dream full of anxiety. She is at the seaside and there is a shark in the water staring at her. While she stares back at it, she realises that she has the same eyes as the shark. She does not have time to fully take this in because the shark approaches with its needle-sharp teeth and devours her.

*   *   *

The patient is attracted to the magnificence of the figure of Mana, who seduces her and leads her to believe that a superior life exists, without limits or everyday frustrations.

She nourishes a feeling of infinite hatred for the world; this is one of the reasons she has become a nocturnal creature that flees the gaze of other human beings. She has constructed an *other reality* where everything is beautiful and delicate, contrasting with the monstrosities and vulgarities of the real world.

However, this withdrawal is not peopled only by idealised figures, but also by dangerous bodies, barbaric female figures full of evil: this is precisely what will trigger the danger of being thoroughly invaded by destructive figures (the witches, incestuous or murderous daughters) with whom Agnese risks fully identifying. Indeed, her dream shows the risk of losing contact with her good parts and being completely swallowed up by a savage animal.

Sexualised withdrawal

A specific characteristic of psychic withdrawal is the capacity to disorientate and ensnare the subject affected by it. An example of this way of operating is clearly described in the dream of a patient focused on the seductive and confusing power of a sexualised withdrawal.

* * *

Twenty-five-year-old Franca came to analysis because she has "numerous emotional problems", among which is her lack of success in having a relationship with a man, even if it is something she wants.

She has never had any important emotive relationships except with a girlfriend or two during adolescence; she confesses that she has a fantasy world peopled with male figures with whom she imagines a wonderful future. For example, she believes that Roberto, a basketball player on the national team, will fall madly in love with her and be the man of her life.

The confusing nature of the withdrawal is revealed in a dream full of anxiety, brought immediately after the beginning of the analysis:

> "There was a young girl in the house of my childhood. I abused her, she touched me and I touched her. Then suddenly she was grown up and wanted to continue, but I told her that it wasn't right, that she would do those things with the person she loved. She replied that there was nothing wrong, it was all OK. I didn't want to and said it was all a mistake . . . it was terrible."

The patient adds that for the whole morning she had been wondering if by chance, when little, she had been abused. Then she intuited that the child in the dream was her. This thing is right inside her.

The interpretation of the dream turns on her fear of being dominated by a force that drives her towards a sexualised withdrawal, a situation that has grown with her since she was little (in the dream, it is her childhood home). She is afraid that this organisation may dominate her and prevent her from having other important relationships.

Franca calms down after this interpretation and adds, "Since I was small I've been precociously fascinated by sexual stimuli . . . at home there were porn mags and I was also aroused by erotic films; then, very early on, I discovered masturbation and I isolated myself. I am very afraid of real contact; I'm frightened of a real relationship. I know that I have to get out of this closed world I shut myself away in where I give myself pleasure, but I'm frightened."

*   *   *

In this patient there is clearly a conflict between the psychopathological construction (the sexualised withdrawal) and the healthier, relational part of the self. In her dream, Franca is afraid that the withdrawal will ensnare and imprison her completely. Even if the masturbatory withdrawal began in childhood as a probable response to an insufficiently receptive environment, this structure has gained in strength over the years and is encroaching on the rest of the self.

In any case, the sexualised withdrawal represents the psychopathological structure at the base of perverse patients' functioning and from which they derive ecstatic sexual pleasure. A situation of this type will be described in the chapter devoted to paedophilia (Chapter Ten). It can also be found, although sporadically, in borderline patients and some psychotics. However, in these cases, the sexualised withdrawal does not represent the hub of the psychopathological state but one of the possible structures that coexists alongside the others. In his book *Sexual States of Mind* (1973), Meltzer recounts many examples of this mental state without, though, indicating that they are part of the psychopathological construction of the psychic withdrawal.

Destructive withdrawal

In destructive withdrawal, the self is dominated by a pathological figure inspired by a delinquent strategy and who is idealised and venerated. The delinquent nucleus wields its power by frightening or seducing the patient with a series of false promises. We saw an example of this in the chapter on psychopathological constructions (Chapter Four): Vittorio revealed to the analyst only after a certain length of time that he identified with the Roman emperor Nero, who justified his violent acts and his claim for destructive revenge.

Another more difficult case is described in the chapter on the perverse fascination of destructiveness (Chapter Thirteen) experienced by Alfredo, a young patient progressively colonised by a type of Nazi homicidal organisation. He fantasised about living in a bunker, operating as a surgeon, excited by the thought of being responsible for the life and death of others. The sight of blood excites him to such an extent he begins to see his own body as an object for torture, slashing and wounding himself.

As I have already mentioned, the destructive organisation is structured like a gang that controls all its members in such a way that they have to actively collaborate and cannot leave the group. When the patient makes a bit of progress, dreams appear that picture his attempts at rebellion together with the retaliation and threats of the gang, often represented as gang of hooligans or a real Mafia-type organisation (Meltzer, 1973; Rosenfeld, 1971).

It is extremely important to understand that the psychic withdrawal of difficult patients is not a static structure but tends to develop and take over the rest of the self. In other words, it is an *intrapsychic delusional structure* that steadily ensnares the healthy part at the expense of a progressive distortion of emotional reality.

The environmental component in the formation of psychotic withdrawal

My hypothesis is that children destined to become psychotic have generally had parents who not only have not known how to emotionally welcome their child's emotional projections, but who, at times, have also invaded the child with their own pathological parts. In this case, the withdrawal is created as a protective defence that tends to exclude any contact with the relational world. In the case of children destined to become psychotic, the withdrawal is the crucible that fuels the psychotic part of the self subsequently destined to colonise the healthy part. I will explain the development of this process better and in more detail in the chapters referring to the psychotic state. What has to be emphasised is that these children construct a parallel sensory reality, an "other world" fuelled by imaginary fantasies, that accompanies them for the whole of their existence and that, in the end, will trigger delusional experiences. In the case of psychotic withdrawal, this is a *secret* place known only to the patient.

The word "dissociation" does not, therefore, imply a vertical split that has occurred within the self, in which one part does not know what the other is concealing, but, on the contrary, the fact that the world of the psychotic withdrawal is nourished only by sensory and imaginary fantasising that never comes into contact with reality. In other words, to use an optical metaphor, it is as though the patient can divide his vision into two: with one eye he can see the construction of the sensory withdrawal, with the other he sees reality; since the two lines of vision never coincide, he never experiences binocular vision, which might lead to insight. The operating of both is kept separate from each other, and they remain parallel without ever meeting. When the patient activates his world of dissociated fantasy, he blocks access to perception of the real world. To use another metaphor, his mind functions like a radio that excludes all other radio stations as soon as it is tuned in to one of them.

In this chapter, I have tried to show how psychic withdrawal is a mental organisation that becomes a constant source of pathology as it accompanies the individual throughout his entire existence. The withdrawal is not just a place in which one can pause to shelter from anxiety, but is, above all, a melting pot that produces alternative realities to the real world. It corresponds to the creation of a sensory and imaginary reality that drains lymph from emotional and psychic development because it shuts down the channels granting passage to experiences useful for growth. The sense of personal identity, particularly, is weakened and deteriorated to varying degrees by the withdrawal, whether this is a collection of pleasurable reveries or takes the extreme forms of a dissociated world as in the psychotic state.

I would now like to say a few words on the stance we should maintain to help the patient get out of his withdrawal.

The patient very rarely communicates the existence of the withdrawal, the sensory fantasies that go with it, and the way he makes use of it to the analyst; indeed, he defends it and cherishes it as a secret and precious place. So, it is up to the analyst's skill to identify its existence and contents with the goal of transforming it. When this process has occurred, the analyst can describe the aims of the withdrawal and show how repeated use of it has a deteriorating effect, something the patient is completely unaware of. Although the patient is *conscious* of having a secret life that unfolds in the withdrawal, he is not *aware* of the destructive effects on his personality. The withdrawal, in fact, sucks his vital energy and damages his emotional development because it offers an easy alternative to the relational world. It is not surprising that, in their external life, these patients seem barely alive, indifferent to what is going on around them, and incapable of carrying through to completion the tasks required of them by daily life. Every undertaking in the real world becomes a source of anxiety for them.

Our analytic work chiefly involves bolstering the patient's awareness, constantly describing to him the dynamics of how the pathogenic part lures him into the withdrawal, cutting him off from his relations and offering him the false advantages of a life dissociated from reality. My clinical experience leads me to believe that intrapsychic interpretations—the ones that describe the dynamics and the reciprocal relationship between the opposing parts of the self—are the most useful in this case for reinforcing the patient's insight. Interpretations of a transferral nature, which bring to light the use the patient makes of the analyst, are obviously important but not as effective for helping the patient become aware of the constant damage he is doing to himself and to his capacity to think. In other words, I treat withdrawal as a drugged structure that drains a person's vitality and sacrifices his emotional growth to the seductive power of sensory pleasure.

I believe that only in this way can a link be established between the healthy part, always in danger of being ensnared and weakened by the enticements offered by the withdrawal, and the analyst's work, which aims to help the patient break free from the confusion and finally be able to make the distinction between what is pleasurable, but turns out to be negative, and what is good and constructive.

CHAPTER SIX

The superego in difficult patients*

"The attitude of the superego should be taken into account –
which has not hitherto been done – in every form of psychical
illness"

(Freud, 1924b, p. 152)

The superego in difficult patients is often tantamount to a negative force, opposing mental growth, which exerts its power
with threats and intimidation. In this case it is a structure that
has inverted its protective function and has been transformed into a
malicious, delusional, or envious figure. While the primitive superego
can gradually be transformed through the analyst accepting it, understanding it, and interpretatively returning it, its pathological organisation requires specific interventions that help clarify to the patient its
nature, its objectives, and its pathogenic action.

In his Los Angeles discussions, Bion (1978, p. 5) notes that one
need only look at a child and say "Ah!" in a reproving way to see him

* Revised and expanded version of a paper originally published in 2002 in Italian, in
Rivista di Psicoanalisi, pp. 517–535. Translated by Philip Slotkin, MA, Cantab. MITI.

wince guiltily before he has any language knowledge whatsoever—or so one would think. He adds that, in order to understand the moral system, we must resort to the term "super-ego", which suggests something above everything else, whereas, in fact, it very probably belongs underneath everything else. In asserting that the power of moral behaviour is based on threats and fear, Bion is drawing attention to the equivocal position of the superego, as both the expression of the moral system and an early organiser of pathology.

The various schools of psychoanalytic theory show differences of emphasis in their view of the function of the superego and of the ego ideal, and their approaches to therapy vary according to their respective hypotheses. In my own opinion, given the origin, meaning, and function of the superego and the ego ideal, both of these entities are readily susceptible to the pathological distortions observed in clinical psychoanalytic work. After all, while we as psychoanalysts are unacquainted with the "normal" superego, we are accustomed to seeing patients with either an abnormal sense of guilt or a seeming absence of guilt.

In this chapter, I shall attempt to describe the forms in which certain pathological aspects of the superego and ego ideal manifest themselves in clinical psychoanalytic work. However, a distinction must first be drawn between the primitive superego and its pathological counterpart. Whereas some clinical situations involve a superego whose primitive aspects feature prominently in the foreground, in other cases one encounters psychopathological structures that do not stem from the primitive superego, even if they share the latter's seductive, dominant, or intimidatory aspects.

The superego between normality and pathology

As a term and a defined entity, the superego was first identified by Freud only in *The Ego and the Id* (1923b), although he had previously described its functions of censorship in dreams, repression, and the unconscious sense of guilt, but without giving them a name. In *The Ego and the Id*, the superego is a psychical agency separate from the ego and having specific relations with the other agencies (the ego and the id) within a tripartite structural division of the psychical apparatus. Freud's 1923 contribution links up with his earlier theoretical model and with the description of the ego ideal given in "On narcissism: an introduction" (1914c). In his treatment of narcissism, Freud attributes to the ego ideal both the state of infantile omnipotence and the alterations in the perception of self and object when one is in love and in the phenomena of collective submission to a leader. In this work, Freud draws a sharp distinction between idealisation and sublimation. Whereas the latter concerns the drive, the former is connected with the object. The ego ideal is an expression of the narcissism that impels the subject to idealise both self and object. Freud shows that the ego ideal forms at the expense of sublimation, which is blocked. Idealisation adversely affects sublimation because the more the ideal aspect comes to the fore, the stronger the demands made on the ego to espouse an ideal and the more the elements of prohibition and criticism are emphasised. In 1923, Freud uses the two terms as synonyms and no longer refers to the ego ideal as an entity separate from and independent of the superego. However, the two terms, superego and ego ideal, are often distinguished and contrasted by the French-speaking psychoanalysts, such as, in particular, Chasseguet-Smirgel (1973). These authors also distinguish between the *ego ideal* and the *ideal ego*, whereas the two entities do not appear as separate concepts in Freud. The ideal ego is a more primitive structure, an expression of narcissism and omnipotence, while the area of the ego ideal retains the characteristics of sublimated ideality and morality. Last, there is the *superego ideal* introduced by Meltzer (1973), which links the ego ideal to the depressive position and is seen as the source of inspiration and creativity.

Since it remains useful for clinical purposes to distinguish between the two terms, I shall consider the pathological transformations of both the ego ideal and the superego.

Freud's theory fails to bridge the gap between the formation of the normal superego and that of its pathological counterpart. In "Mourning and melancholia" (1917e), he refers to a conscience imbued with powerful sadism that gives rise to an intrapsychic vicious circle, but in *The Ego and the Id* (1923b) he describes instead a superego that is formed by the introjection of parental images and becomes the representative of all value judgements. A polarity in the conception of the superego remains apparent throughout Freud's complex construction: on the one hand, it is seen as the expression of sociality and of positive identifications with the father figure, while,

on the other, it is the heir to the cannibalistic destructiveness of melancholia.

The importance of the aggressive instinct is implicit in Freud's
conception of superego pathology: he writes that in melancholia the
superego is "as it were, a pure culture of the death instinct" (1923b,
p. 53); while later, in "The economic problem of masochism" (1924c),
he notes that owing to defusion of the death instinct, the superego
becomes cruel and inexorable against the ego. In *Civilization and Its
Discontents* (1930a), the aggression of the superego is said to be
turned against the ego itself and transformed into the sense of guilt.
Considering all these facts, Freud notes that the severity of the superego no longer coincides with that of the real parents, but depends
instead on a combination of environmental and innate constitutional
factors.

Taking as her starting point Freud's analysis of the process of
melancholia, Melanie Klein states that the infantile superego is essentially sadistic and postulates that this is due to the cruelty and pitilessness of the first introjections. Hence, the principal aim in child
analysis is, in her view, to make the superego more benevolent and
not to reinforce it as advocated by Anna Freud (Klein, 1927a). The
superego does not coincide with the introjection of the parents, but
arises spontaneously out of the child's sadistic fantasies (Klein, 1927b).
In the paranoid–schizoid position, the superego is itself the bad object
that must be destroyed by all possible means.

Klein (1963) lays no particular emphasis on the ideal ego and holds
that the ego ideal is the ideal, omnipotent part of the self, a concept
advanced by Freud before he developed his ideas on the superego.
She sees the idealisation of the object as a defence against persecution,
fusion with the idealised object being an initial defence against annihilation anxiety.

Klein's innovation was to link the nature of the primitive superego
to the destructive instinct. A depressed patient's sense of guilt is attributed to the excess of unconscious hate and the awareness that this hate
might destroy the object (Klein, 1935). Part of the guilt is due to the
object's ideal demands: objects are either extremely bad or utterly
perfect; in other words, the loved objects are intensely moral and
demanding (Klein, 1948). The primitive superego is born of the death
instinct and of the violence that is inflicted by the child on frustrating
objects and by which the child feels threatened. While, on the one

hand, the primitive superego perpetuates cruelty, on the other its introjection of the good object will constitute its benevolent aspect.

Freud, too, describes the protective aspect of the superego, which he connects with the love of the parents. At the end of his essay "Humour" (1927d), he notes that the fact that the superego tries to console the ego and to protect it from suffering does not contradict its origins in the parental agency.[5]

Pathology of the superego

The superego in melancholia

According to Freud (1917e) and Abraham (1973[1924]), a melancholic's perception of not being loved gives rise to a constant reproach to the love object, which is accused of inadequacy and unworthiness. This forms the basis of a sadomasochistic type of object relationship, in which the sadistic aspect is manifested in repeated accusations of imperfection directed at the object, while the masochistic side consists in adopting the position of an unhappy victim: the melancholic tortures the object, by which he in turn feels tortured. This unhappy object relationship reflects an inner conflict between the patient's superego and ego, in which the superego accuses the ego of unworthiness, while the ego in turn attacks the superego for its harshness.

This kind of pathology can be illustrated by the following case history.

*   *   *

The female patient in question, aged forty-eight at the beginning of her analysis, has already had a period of psychotherapy and a previous analysis that was broken off after two years. She has been admitted to hospital several times for depression, on one occasion having received ECT. She tells me this only after the analysis has begun. She is married with one child. She lives with her husband, with whom she has not had an affective relationship for some time. Sexual relations have ceased at his instigation. Her resentment towards her husband seems to be masked by a sense of superiority and contempt.

On commencing her analysis, the patient appears to harbour the perception of being unable to face the second part of her life because she feels threatened by a profound sense of destruction and persecution. This inner situation is graphically illustrated by the first dreams she brings to the analysis: for instance,

> "In a Mediterranean town, I am arrested and accused of being dressed too smartly; I am on a road that leads off to somewhere unknown . . . there is one last building and a church, but in fact only the façade of the church exists, like in a stage set."

The church is associated with the one where she was married, and the town is where she went on honeymoon.

A few months into her analysis, the patient discovers that her husband is having an affair with another woman, and feels compelled, albeit against her will, to separate from him when she realises that he has no intention of ending it. It is during this period that violent feelings of jealousy and resentment come up. In this situation, the patient feels herself to be a "victim of her husband", but fails to admit to even the slightest responsibility on her own part for the failure of the marriage. She has completely blotted out any awareness of her own infidelities, which have punctuated the couple's marriage from its earliest years.

It is not long before a sadomasochistic relationship arises in the transference, too. The patient accuses me of numerous deficiencies, cruelties, and omissions, often directing vehement "indictments" at me. I am the butt of constant disputes about session times, holidays, and the price of her sessions, to the extent that at one point she even claims to be "resolved to protect myself better in my next analysis"! According to the patient, my analytic behaviour is an ongoing exercise in cruelty: if I do not interpret it is because I want to humiliate her, but if I do it is with the aim of making her feel awful. I, the analyst, want to deprive her of her pleasures, of her relationships with her partner or with other men she happens to meet, and I will end up making her live a monastic life.

The patient manifestly maintains a relationship of extreme cruelty with the object, which, at the same time, she holds responsible for her sadism (the object being myself in the analysis, and the members of her family in her life outside the consulting room).

In the countertransference, I observe in myself an unusual level of difficulty in sympathising with, and having warm feelings towards, her, and I become aware of the risk of the analytic relationship repeating the "models" of the patient's life so far, with her parents in her childhood and with her husband later—a life analysed in predominantly negative terms.

This relational situation is mirrored in the patient's internal world, which includes a parent who constantly accuses her of being a good-for-nothing, and is bound up with her relationship with her father in infancy, when he was experienced as the only one of her parents to deserve respect.

She remembers her father as a very severe person, and in her internal world he charges her with being utterly incapable and lacking in any personal qualities. However, the patient says, this father has an Achilles heel: he wants to engage in sexual activity with her. On this foundation, she establishes a defence of sexual seduction against the cruelty of the superego, but this defence fails to change the quality of the relationship with her internal object, for seduction is always followed by an exacerbation of the superego's never-ending accusations that she is "nothing but a whore . . ."[6] The superego object is contradictory and confusing—it exalts her and makes her feel special, only to attack and denigrate her afterwards—thus causing her to feel uncertain and mixed up.

This atmosphere, with its mixture of excitation, persecution, and projected guilt, gradually dissipates. As she begins to have a better subjective relationship with the world, no longer always feeling envious and full of destructive wishes, she has the following dream:

> "I look at my hands and notice that my ring finger, which was broken, has healed, leaving a scar."

She associates to her brother, who had had a finger amputated after a wartime bomb found in the garden went off. Identified with her brother, the patient is telling herself in the dream that something has after all remained and that she can still use her other fingers. She also associates to her failed marriage and the emergence of friendlier feelings towards her husband.

In addition, this phase sees the appearance of regret at what she has lost in her past life—because a "false and capricious" part held sway over her—and the possibility of taking a more balanced view in which she can make better use of what she has. After the fifth year of analysis, this new constructive atmosphere is confirmed both in her relationships outside the consulting room and in the analytic communication.

* * *

This clinical account clearly illustrates the constant exchange of accusations between the superego, the patient, and her object. From the very first dream, a connection can be traced between accusation and guilt (being "dressed too smartly" and the narcissistic choice in her relationships and marriage).

Notwithstanding some difficult analytic transactions, this case seems likely to have a favourable outcome (as, in fact, it eventually did).

The destructive superego organisation

"In other situations the connection between guilt and sin is less obvious: the superego is transformed by the establishment of a narcissistic and destructive organization into a 'pure culture of the death instinct'" (Freud, 1923b, p. 53).

* * *

The following brief account concerns a woman doctor, aged about thirty-five, who requests a consultation on the possibility of analytic therapy, a choice about which she is very uncertain. Some years ago, she lapsed into a depression, which she confronts by an alcohol dependency that enables her to carry on working somehow or other. She has three older brothers and was born when her parents were already advanced in years; her father, with whom she recalls having had a warm relationship when she was small, died of a heart attack when she was only seven years old. Her mother did not tell her at the time that he had died; when she asked why he was not there she was told that he had gone on a trip to America. It was not until a few months later that one of the nuns at her school took it upon herself to tell her the truth, at the same time impressing on her the importance of being a good girl so as not to upset her mother.

At the two initial interviews, the patient says that she would like to die and that she finds it hard to imagine that something like psychoanalysis can help her. The main reason for her depression is that the man with whom she had hoped for a permanent relationship has left her. Having always seen herself as an insignificant person, the patient feels that she has no hope of finding another partner. In the first interview, her situation seems to me particularly serious, partly because of her explicit aspiration to end her life, but I am somewhat relieved by our second meeting, when she appears slightly calmer and tells me she has opted to commence analytic treatment.

However, she fails to turn up for her third appointment. When I phone her home to enquire why she has not come, her mother tells me she has attempted suicide by taking a drug overdose and has been taken in a coma to the hospital's resuscitation ward. Two weeks later, she phones me from the psychiatric clinic to which she has been admitted and asks whether I am still available to begin analysis with her.

The reasons for the suicide attempt are the first aspect to be explored in the analysis. The patient explains her plunge towards death as just desserts for the failure of her life. During the analysis, I discover that whenever any difficulty arises, an inner voice tells her that she is incapable of anything and has no right to exist in the world. This superego voice stems from a highly structured narcissistic organisation that opposes any perception of need or suffering and demands eradication of the weak. If she were to express suffering or ask for help, she would be attacked. It is, indeed, precisely at the moment when the patient asks for help and entrusts herself to analysis that her superego, which insists on sacrifice, becomes most dangerous. That is what occurred after the first two interviews when the hope of being helped by analysis came up.

In the transference, the patient seems totally docile; she expresses neither recriminations nor complaints, is never aggressive, and tends not to suffer consciously at separations, which are dealt with by acceptance of the object's complete disappearance. This passive acceptance of the experience of abandonment seems to be connected with repeated actual traumatic experiences in infancy. At any rate, the perception of need must be obliterated because it is a source of pain to which no response can be forthcoming. I postulate that the patient has internalised a depressed mother who imbues neediness with guilt and demands independence and self-sufficiency based on "moral" imperatives.

* * *

The narcissistic organisation, which punishes need and any request for help, possesses the character of an ideal superego with a destructive potential that is not perceived as such by the patient. A significant part of the analytic work consisted of laying bare the power of this organisation and progressively reducing its hegemony. Note that, in terms of technique, it is essential to begin by removing the patient from the sway of the pathological organisation, as any interpretation would otherwise risk being distorted and swallowed up by the destructive superego.

Pathology of the ego ideal

"Benign" narcissism

Any discussion of ideals and idealisation inevitably calls to mind the relevant contributions of Winnicott (1971) and Kohut (1971), because these authors, despite their differing models and sources of inspiration, opened up new perspectives on the structuring role played by processes of idealisation. Both hold that children, at an early stage of development, need to experience the illusion of positive omnipotence and, by idealisation of self and object, to structure the sense of individuality and of personal significance.

As we know, these insights have not only helped us to gain a better understanding of certain phases of primitive development, but also led to changes in technique based—especially in the Kohut school—on exploiting aspects of narcissistic relationships. In day-to-day clinical practice, we have come to attach more importance to primitive idealising transferences, these being seen as possible staging posts on the way to a more mature and integrated object relationship.

The second part of my contribution will be devoted to exemplifying the role of idealisation, seen as a transitional phase from an infantile relational world to a more mature object relationship. At the same time, I shall seek to distinguish this mental state from that of the kind of narcissistic idealisation that favours idol formation.

*   *   *

A twenty-one-year-old male patient comes into analysis owing to a state of deep distress exacerbated by the break-up of a relationship; he finds himself unable to study and is using soft drugs. After a difficult beginning to the analysis, his condition improves so that he is able to resume his studies, the improvement being accompanied by a positive, idealised attachment to me.

The dreams from this period feature beautiful tropical forests, brilliantly coloured plants, and prehistoric animals (mammoths). In these dreams, plants and animals vanish suddenly and mysteriously, as if swallowed up in the void. The associations to the material, which suggest a personification of the beauty of nature, reveal an idealising infantile passion that impels the patient to embrace objects that prove to be ephemeral and transitory.

Narcissistic fusion and the relationship between idealisation and falsification are described in a dream whose subject is the fascination of beauty. In the dream, the patient is blinded by a very beautiful woman who gently seduces him; he lets himself be blinded, but then notices that he can see; to be able to go on seeing at least a little, he knows he must not tell this to the woman.

The experience depicted in the dream is neither destructive nor perverse, but ultimately betrays a dangerous limitation of perception. The patient avoids this risk by removing himself from the total dominion of the fascinating image, which would blind him completely.

*   *   *

I believe that this patient is describing a distortion in the enjoyment of beauty connected with narcissistic identification. The blinding alludes to the power of an object that can enrapture and transform perception: the ideal becomes narcissistic idealisation in order to satisfy the need for fusion with an object felt to be desirable and superior.

This last point leads us conveniently to the problems presented by the constitution of the idol.

Formation of the idol

The idol not only does not represent a continuation of the ideal but is, in fact, a pathological distortion of it. This is illustrated by the following example of a thirty-year-old male patient, a sadomasochistic, homosexual paedophile who is attracted to children or, more often, male adolescents. In this fragment, I shall disregard all the sadomasochistic aspects with their inevitable transference and countertransference implications, and concentrate on the paedophilic nucleus, which, in the eyes of the patient, possesses the status of a real world and the quality of an idol to be venerated.

*   *   *

Michele[7] was an intelligent and precocious child who grew up in a state of affective remoteness from his father, whose harshness and authoritarianism he always hated, while enjoying a privileged relationship of mutual seduction with his mother.

Spending much of his day in groups of adolescents, he is irresistibly attracted by the boys' bodies, legs as shown off by their shorts, silken hair, and smooth skin. For him the sight of an adolescent boy is an occasion for pleasure, a unique experience which must be grasped and which appears all the more inviting because it is signalled by the youngster himself, who, in the eyes of the patient, radiates the pleasure of sexuality acted out with his coevals. In order not to be excluded from a relationship with the boys, which he experiences as life-giving, the patient makes sure of being with them as much as possible. The company of people of his own age arouses no curiosity or desire in him, and, in particular, is not a moral imperative, as in the case of the boys.

Just before the summer holidays in the third year of his analysis, the patient brings an anxiety dream:

> he is sitting on the lap of a young man called Mario in a climate of erotic and playful intimacy. Mario gradually moves away from him and disappears. The patient feels lonely and desperate. He feels that he is responsible for Mario's disappearance: he ought to have taken more care of him and devoted all his energy to him so as to keep him by his side.

He feels that the blame for his undoing is entirely his own. Mario, the patient says, is wise; he knows the secret of life and how to be happy. He thinks Mario could have made him happy. He himself is to blame because he failed to take care of him at all times. Anxiety is mixed with guilt.

Inwardly ruling out an interpretation concerning the forthcoming separation from the analysis (a holiday period is imminent), I consider the context of the dream and the paedophilic universe that reigns over the patient's mind. In his internal world, what sustains him is the boy-idol-object, and not the analyst or his parents. The dream actually portrays the experience of anxiety when the delusional illusion of the idol disappears. The idol, according to the dream, demands total submission and devotion, and if the patient loses it he is plunged into unhappiness and guilt. The idol surrounds itself with a myth. In the patient's fantasy, the "boy" is the idol to be venerated. In the dream, the illusion of complete happiness in the veneration of the boy-idol abandons him and the ideal world now inspires guilt.

* * *

The formation of the idol, a pathogenic structure, is very remote from idealisation. In this case, the patient idolises a fetish-object which takes the form of an a-relational world (in which sexualised pleasure continues to play an important part) that promises superiority over need and over the everyday experience of life. Involving as it does the negation of time, ageing, and death, the repudiation of reality in paedophilia assumes the character of delusional fascination and is the precondition for entry into an illusory world that leads directly, by way of sexual attraction, to incest and perversion.

Whereas idealisation has to do with love, albeit a primitive love, the idol is venerated for reasons of power. For this reason, it, in turn, demands and obtains submission. The collusion between the idol and the ego is explained by the promise of pleasure and well-being emanating from the idol.

An idol assumes power over the personality by first bewitching and then dominating it. The idol results from a falsification in which a seductive element—power or superiority—is idealised; in dynamic terms, it can be seen as a split-off, anti-emotional part of the patient that confuses him and promises paradise if he subjects himself to the boys. Such cases involve a delusional construction in which insight lacks the strength to penetrate and collides with the barrier of a psychotic thought.

A long period of analytic work was required before the patient was enabled to "see" the illusory construction without still being blinded by, and dependent on, it. For this point to be reached, it was necessary progressively to forge a relational and emotional world that strength-ened the patient and released him from the sway of the idol's illusory promises.

The perversion of the superego

It is important to note that psychoanalysis has, from the beginning, demonstrated the existence of two types of superego, the first of which can, for the sake of simplicity, be called *oedipal*, while the second belongs to the psychopathology of melancholia. According to Freud, the normal, or oedipal, superego results from the overcoming of infantile omnipotence as a child gradually comes to accept the regulating and protective function of the father. The melancholic superego, on the other hand, falls from the beginning within the traumatic experience of the relationship with the mother.

In "Mourning and melancholia", Freud (1917e, p. 249) writes,

> An object-choice, an attachment of the libido to a particular person, had at one time existed; then, owing to *a real slight* or disappointment coming from this loved person, the object relationship was shattered. ... Thus the shadow of the object fell upon the ego, and the latter could henceforth be judged by a special agency, as though it were an object, the forsaken object. In this way an object-loss was transformed into an ego-loss and the conflict between the ego and the loved person into a cleavage between the critical activity of the ego and the ego as altered by identification.

Hence, the critical aspect of the superego arises from trauma. For a pathological superego to form, the trauma must be an early one and must coincide with the primitive character of the relationship. This point is emphasised by Abraham (1973[1924]) in his chapter on melancholia, where he stresses the importance of the soil on which the trauma falls and the child's need for love in order to overcome hate. Hatred of the disappointing object pervades the melancholic superego, and the early nature of the trauma coincides with the primitiveness of the object-relations situation.

Thus far, Freud and Abraham. In the subsequent vision of Klein, the primitive superego and the pathological superego increasingly merge, owing to the decline in the importance of the maternal trauma to which Freud drew attention and which was emphasised by Abraham. It is Klein who postulated that the more severe and pitiless the superego, the more primitive it is.

By laying stress on the kinship between pathology and primitive states of mind, Klein's model links the pitilessness of the superego with the level of aggression present in the primitive ego. Klein holds that the struggle against the superego, the first bad object, commences early on: fearing punishment and revenge, the child hates and is afraid of the mother, who is experienced as an ultra-severe superego. In Klein's view, only the stable introjection of the good object can diminish its implacability and harshness.

Observing which superego a melancholic patient has at his disposal, by what judge or "morality" he is judged, and what "good" object sustains him (an object that is, moreover, venerated and loved), we are bound to consider that this object is perfect and implacable. By demanding that the ego itself be ideal, the pathological superego maintains an implacability towards ambivalent aspects of the ego, which are not tolerated. Much of the veneration and fear of the ideal object is due to the threat of unhappiness and the imminence of punishment.

It follows that a child can gain access to the oedipal experience only after elaborating and transforming the persecutory, threatening superego. Failing this process, the child will be unable to internalise the ordering paternal function that characterises the oedipal superego described by Freud.

However, primitiveness and pitilessness are not the only aspects of the complex pathology of the superego. Albeit not explicitly, the element of trauma reappears in post-Kleinian theories in the guise of an affective trauma due to the lack of an empathic response from the primary object: some of the relevant authors emphasise the failure of the first object relations rather than primitiveness.

Bion (1959) considers that the mother's systematic rejection of the child's projective identification gives rise to a superego that is intrinsically hostile to curiosity and to infantile vitality, while Rosenfeld (1971) describes the destructive narcissism that dominates the healthy part of the personality by virtue solely of the force of idealised, "moral" propaganda. In these cases, the experience of growth mediated by a good relationship is lacking and the personality is colonised by a pathological structure.

The ideal object present in the pathological superego gives rise to a narcissistic type of morality—a "moral narcissism"—in which, on the basis of the veneration of a state of "superiority", identification with the ideal object leads to a pathological sense of guilt. From this point of view, morality is nothing but the cruelty that worms its way into the ideal object, resulting in a practical morality based on submission to, and veneration of, the "moral", ideal object.

The pathological organisation of the superego, considered in these terms, thus corresponds to its deadliness and not to its primitive character. It is less a matter of primitive pitilessness ("an eye for an eye, a tooth for a tooth") than of perversion and intimidatory propaganda on the part of the "moral" agency.

This suggests the existence of a superego that has no interest in establishing guilt or inflicting punishment, but, instead, seeks to seduce or intimidate in order to subjugate and distort mental growth. The superego and the ego ideal are then no longer internal objects, however primitive, but psychopathological structures that wield power over the rest of the personality.

In this contribution, I have sought to show that pathology of the superego and of the ego ideal does not coincide with primitiveness, but takes the form of specific types of organisation of the mind, tantamount to pathological structures that are ensconced within the personality and possess special power because they are valued and venerated. For clinical purposes, these pathological organisations must be seen as structures that do not represent continuations of either the normal or the primitive superego.

It is useful to invoke not only the superego, but also the ego ideal to explain the magnetic attraction and euphoria stemming from the power of the idol over the rest of the personality.[8] For this reason, it is, in my view, better to refer to a pathological organisation of the ego ideal than to pathology of the ego ideal. This is the case where the pathology, while resulting from the primal trauma, loses its connection with it and is fuelled by new constructions. Promising salvation at the cost of perverting the perception of human reality, the idol becomes what can only be described as a pathological organisation.

It is not unusual to observe the normal superego, the primitive superego, and the superego resulting from the psychopathological structure all operating at the same time at different levels and in different areas in one and the same patient. While the primitive superego can be transformed gradually by the analyst's acceptance, comprehension, and interpretative responses, the pathological organisation can be neither integrated nor transformed, but must, like a delusional formation, be *deconstructed* so as progressively to reduce its power over the rest of the personality.

Superego psychopathological constructions

To understand the genesis of the most serious distortions of the super-ego and the ego ideal, it is, therefore, necessary to consider the mental structures that originate from early traumatic areas and develop in isolation and lack of relationship. The superego derived from the des-tructive organisation is, as shown in my second clinical example, one that is structured in the absence of internal parents and expresses a narcissistic hatred of need and dependence. These unelaborated areas become psychic structures—virtual "neo-creations"—in which aggression, seduction, terror, and fascination hold sway. Structures of this kind may be said to have developed *instead of the superego and ego ideal*, so that they are unable to grow into more mature forms as in the case of primitive formations.

Genetically, the psychopathological superego structures are very different from primitive superego structures. Although the terms "pathological" and "primitive" are often used synonymously in tradi-tional psychoanalytic theory, the two distinct territories of primitive-ness and pathology are often confused because they both involve elements of splitting, idealisation, concreteness, and grandiosity. Psy-chopathological organisations, however, unlike primitive structures, are totally lacking in the quality of development (Caper, 1998). If the distinction is not made, one loses sight of the negative force that oppo-ses mental growth and stems from psychopathological superego structures that impose their will by intimidation and the illusion of well-being.

In extreme pathological organisations, the personality is subordi-nated to a criminal or psychotic superego nucleus that holds it in thrall, perverting the conscience (superego) and distorting ideals (ego ideal).

In some anorexic or psychotic patients there is no difference between the superego and idealisation of their own physical and mental self-annihilation (De Masi, 1996). The superego's dependence on the destructive part of the personality impels the individual to embrace non-life-affirming goals disguised by "moral" precepts. In this way, the pathological forces progressively dissolve the relation-ship with a human object, and construct in its place psychic struc-tures—the psychopathological organisations—that generate illusions in the patient, who is, thereby, seduced and captured by the promise of omnipotence. In seriously disturbed mental states, such as anorexia, drug addiction, or perversions, the idols gain power over the personality by first bewitching it and then brutally dominating it. As the post-Kleinian authors (for example, Meltzer, 1973; Rosenfeld, 1971) have often pointed out, this type of pathological organisation may be represented in dreams by a criminal gang that dominates and terrifies the patient: the idol is, after all, the fruit of falsification and intimidatory propaganda.

In such a case, it is hard to tell whether this is due to perversion of the moral agency or to pathological structures that have taken the place of the superego. The fact that every perverse system assumes the form of a hyper-moral organisation and that, conversely, the superego tends to destroy life in every hyper-moral system explains the paradoxical nature of morality and confirms the kinship between the superego and destructiveness in psychopathological structures.

CHAPTER SEVEN

The unconscious in neurotic, borderline, and psychotic patients*

"In that period, practically all my life was lived not as life as such, but as a film or a mirror of the film that my mind was projecting on to the screen of my unconscious. Unfortunately, the unconscious only feels and doesn't see, just as the eyes only see and don't feel . . ."

(A patient describing a psychotic episode
that occurred during analysis)

Much contemporary research has stressed the importance—for the structuring of the self—of the earliest mother–infant interrelations that occur during the first months of life and that are located on a pre-symbolic level. These mimicking, visual, and gesturing exchanges are considered fundamental for the formation of the very first elements that will lay the basis for the child's unconscious emotional life. The unconscious system is not a given fact from

---

* A shorter version of this paper was first presented at the International Psychoanalytical Association Congress in Mexico City in August 2011. Translated by Philip Slotkin, MA, Cantab. MITI.

the beginning, but develops if the necessary emotive conditions exist for its initial founding and growth. Absence of these conditions causes irreversible damage to the good psychic functioning of the individual. My hypothesis is that at the base of the most difficult psychopathologies there is a deterioration of the unconscious emotional–receptive functions.

Psychoanalysis as a research method and a therapy (the Freudian *Iunktim*) is based on the discovery of the function of the dynamic unconscious, a structured and complex system that, in the course of a psychic conflict, is capable of repressing and removing from awareness affects or emotions that are incompatible with consciousness.

The interpretative work, by offering the analysand the possibility of understanding what has been repressed, restores the lost meaning of wishes, thoughts, or impulses and, therefore, it strengthens the ego.

In this chapter, I will explore at greater depth the difficulties that emerge with patients who have not developed the necessary intuitive–emotional capacities for understanding themselves and who are not capable of containing or working through their emotions. These patients are generically termed *serious* because they do not respond to the common analytic approach and fall outside the model based on the functioning of the laws of the dynamic unconscious.

Is it possible to establish a correlation between different levels of pathology and the distortions of some unconscious functions necessary for good mental functioning?

My hypothesis is that mental health depends on the possibility of using an apparatus that allows us to contain and keep our emotions alive as well as to give meaning to our existence. This apparatus functions all the time, beyond individual consciousness. Some patients have this apparatus or, at least, are in the condition to develop it, whereas others seem to be lacking it completely.

Although the criteria of accepting a patient in analysis have changed, the notion of analysability—an important topic of debate in the past—has its roots in this difference.

I start from the premise that the unconscious has been conceptualised in different ways in the various analytic models—for example, those proposed by Freud, Klein, or Bion—and that every model applies to a specific clinical situation and to a specific unconscious function.

I shall now summarise the views on the unconscious offered by these authors. My elementary account does not do justice to the complexity and depth of these authors' ideas; I limit myself to comparing the various approaches with a view to highlighting the differences rather than to discussing and analysing in depth the individual models.[9]

Freud's dynamic unconscious

Freud uses the term "unconscious" to refer to two different kinds of psychic experiences of which the subject is unaware: preconscious thought processes that have easy access to consciousness, and those that can be recovered only with great difficulty and belong to the unconscious proper. From a descriptive viewpoint, there are two types of unconscious, though in dynamic terms there is only one (Freud, 1923b).

Topically, the term "unconscious" refers to a system of the psychic apparatus composed of contents that have been denied access to the preconscious–conscious system by means of repression; the objects are conserved as unconscious representations linked by mnemonic remnants.

The Freudian unconscious is, therefore, a psychic locus having specific mechanisms and contents. The latter are the "unmasked" drives, instincts, and affects governed by the primary process, by condensation, and by displacement, and are recognisable only through the derivatives that gain access to the preconscious–conscious systems as compromising formations deformed by censure.

The unconscious is the reservoir of primitive wishes and instincts from the personal and phylogenetic past, but is also the locus of the primal fantasies that structure the subject's infantile experiences; these fantasies are unconscious mental representations of the drives.

The first split between the unconscious and preconscious is effected by infantile repression. The characteristics of the unconscious system are those of the primary system: absence of denial and doubt, indifference to reality, regulation on the basis of the pleasure–unpleasure principle.

In Freud's second topography, the unconscious comprises not only the id, but also part of the ego and superego. Repression is not the only mechanism that gives rise to the unconscious; many other ways exist. Splitting, negation, and denial are defence mechanisms that

support and mediate the conflicts between the various psychic structures, or between the ego and reality, and participate in forming the
unconscious since they themselves are unconscious mechanisms. In
perversion, for example, splitting of the ego leads to two opposing
ideas of reality coexisting, each unaware of the other.

Alongside the dynamic unconscious, whose basis is repression and
the conflict between instinct and culture, Freud described other forms
of unconscious functioning. In *The Ego and the Id* (Freud, 1923b), he
writes that, whereas it is true that everything repressed is unconscious, not all the unconscious coincides with the repressed. A portion
of the ego, too, is unconscious—not in the sense that it is preconscious,
but that it belongs to the non-repressed unconscious. While having the
highly evolved unconscious functions of emotional communication in
mind, Freud (1912b, 1915e) does not coherently develop these ideas,
and neither, for a long time, will others after him. Instead, in analytic
theory, emphasis is given to the repressed unconscious, anchored to
animal legacy as presented in *Civilization and Its Discontents* (Freud,
1930a), which considers mankind's unhappiness to be a consequence
of the irreconcilable difference between nature and culture.

The Kleinian unconscious

Klein accepted Freud's theory of the unconscious but contributed two
significant innovations: the notion of unconscious phantasy and the
introduction of the concept of splitting of the object and, later, of splitting and projection (projective identification). In her theory, unconscious phantasy differs from unconscious representation. It is not only
the psychic representative of the drive but also a mental representation that includes physical perceptions interpreted as relations
between objects, and the corresponding anxieties and defences. The
Kleinian unconscious is made up of relations between internal objects
perceived concretely, and phantasies about them (Isaacs, 1952).

The phantasies may be elaborated or modified by manipulation of
the body (masturbatory phantasies), or produced actively through
the imagination; they are unconscious because, in line with Freud's
thinking, they cannot be known directly, but only through the clinical
material (the interpretation of tics, phantasies, and games). Relations
and the significance of the mental objects (good and bad)—according

to the quality of the physical sensations—are structured in the unconscious phantasy through splitting.

The spatial metaphor is emphasised in Klein's description of the unconscious: in projective identification, unwanted contents, including parts of the self banished from consciousness, are projected outside, deposited in and confused with an object, and subsequently reintrojected. Furthermore, with projective identification, the concept of unconscious broadens to include the two-person sphere: the projection that occurs within another person modifies the perception of the subject projecting and distorts the perception of the object receiving the projection.

Bion's unconscious

In Bion, the unconscious forfeits the ontic connotation of place: it is a function of the mind and not a space for depositing the repressed. So, when we are walking, we are conscious of doing so, but we are not aware of the operations that we carry out in order to walk; if we were, our mind would be crowded with perceptions and we would not be free to walk.

The contact barrier and the *alpha function* serve to free and transform the mind of an excess of sensory stimuli. Dreams are the psyche's *modus operandi* in life: their function is to establish the contact barrier through which *beta* elements are transformed into *alpha* elements and sensations become emotions. At the beginning of life, this function is performed by the mother through her capacity for reverie. The concept of repression is replaced by a semi-permeable membrane, a kind of unconscious organ of consciousness, which allows the processing and knowledge of the world and emotions.

The clash is not between the repressed (Freud) or the split unconscious (Klein) and consciousness, but between waking and sleeping, between aware and unaware consciousness. The unconscious is a metaboliser of psychic experiences, and, if it does not function satisfactorily, the mind will be unable to produce thoughts (the semi-permeable membrane and the alpha function).

The patient can be conscious, but not aware, thanks to the theory of thoughts without a thinker. In addition, for Bion, "thinking" coincides with the possibility of "dreaming": dreaming is a process whereby the unconscious becomes conscious and is also the means for passing from the paranoid–schizoid position (expulsion) to the depressive position (assimilation). Preverbal unconscious material must be submitted constantly to dreamwork, which acts outside consciousness. The dream, like the unconscious, is an intrapyshic and interrelational communication; it is a function that moulds and records emotions, an ever-present daily activity (Bion, 1992).

A patient

Anna, aged twenty-five, enters analysis because she is tormented by panic attacks and continuous hypochondriac experiences that lead to frequent, urgent hospitalisations. Her having been recently abandoned by her boyfriend, and especially her father's death, about a year ago, seem to be the events that have shattered her vitality and pleasure in life. It seems odd that Anna, the only child in her family, who was deeply loved by her father and was a very bright and courageous girl, has gone through such a collapse. But a dream in the first months of analysis clarifies the reasons for her breakdown. In the dream, she represents herself as a tourist guide who is brilliantly describing in detail the monuments in a square. However, in the dream, Anna is aware that she has never been in that city and does not know anything about the monuments she is talking about.

*   *   *

Grotstein (1981) states that dreams perform a fundamentally important function in allowing psychic life to be observed and understood. For this to happen, however, an unseen observer must be present to annotate the plot and verify and validate its truths and messages. The dreamer who dreams a dream and the one who understands it may together be deemed a unit that maintains the stability of the sense of personal identity, by constantly integrating emotional experience and conferring meaning on it. The dreamer who understands the dream is the representation of an intuitive internalised function, which picks up the narrative significance and integrates the story so that it becomes possible to understand it.

It is easy to assume that, to construct a dream of this kind, Anna needs to have both functions: being able both to "dream"—that is, to formulate thoughts that represent it—and to understand these thoughts with hindsight.

In the dream, Anna sees herself engaged in producing an idealised self-image before the group of tourists (her parents and, in the transference, the analyst), but, in fact, she "knows" she is showing false knowledge. The dream talks to the dreamer and tells her that in her life she has managed to deceive herself as a grown-up, without having actually developed a real-life experience. Anna seems to unconsciously intuit a psychic truth concerning herself, about which she can now become aware. In this patient there seems to be an ability to "see" a core of truth that enables her to understand what might be the grounds of her suffering. In other words, the unconscious talks to the patient with the language of psychic truth. The therapeutic issue consists in evaluating, moment by moment, what degree of truth the patient is able to recognise (Money-Kyrle, 1968).

The emotional–receptive unconscious

Psychoanalytic therapy treats all the mental operations (constructed over time and governed by the primary affective bonds) that organise our processes for knowing and relate us to the world. It makes use of a natural psychic function, in other words, the *emotional–intuitive* function that is capable of observing its own mental processes. These unconscious functions are potentially present in every human being, except when distorted or weakened in those cases of psychic illness.

One of the most significant contributions made by contemporary psychoanalysis has shown us that intuitive–emotional thought develops only if the child receives empathic responses from the primary object; I am referring to the receptiveness and to the restitution by the maternal figure of his first communicative projections. Thanks to being treated as a person, the child is gradually inserted into the human world of meanings, and is able to become, in his turn, a person capable of conferring meaning on his own experiences, of understanding his fellow beings, and of communicating with them (Bordi, 2009).

The psychoanalytic process can, therefore, be defined as a method for developing the intuitive–emotional faculties. The analyst must have the capacity for *reverie*, or, in other words, appropriately use his own intuitive imagination to understand his own and the other's emotions. This constant intuitive exploration constitutes the setting, an experimental field that is suitable for the development of the patient's potential faculties of insight.

In my view, the function that allows unconscious perception of one's internal world belongs to an emotional–receptive unconscious, the same unconscious that Freud described, but never completely finished theorising, in his work "Recommendations to physicians practising psycho-analysis" (1912e). Here, he says that the analyst

> must turn his own unconscious like a receptive organ towards the transmitting unconscious of the patient. He must adjust himself to the patient as a telephone receiver is adjusted to the transmitting microphone. Just as the receiver converts back into sound waves the electric oscillations in the telephone line which were set up by sound waves, so the doctor's unconscious is able, from the derivatives of the unconscious which are communicated to him, to reconstruct that unconscious, which has determined the patient's free associations. (Freud, 1912e, p. 114)

With these statements, Freud, in my opinion, anticipates some concepts of contemporary psychoanalysis that are concerned with the unaware components of emotional perception and of the self's unconscious roots.

Emde (1989), for example, describes an affective "pre-representative centre" of the self that originates from early experiences with the mother (found also in various other lives and cultures) and that guarantees a sensation of the continuity of the self during development despite the ongoing changes we are all subject to.

Stolorow and Atwood (1992) broaden the concept of the unconscious to include that part of the personal story that, never having been confirmed, cannot become a conscious experience. These authors postulate that not only the omnipotent and destructive parts are rendered unconscious, but also the good and constructive impulses when they conflict with the views of the person looking after the child; in this way, a large part of infantile awareness and "wisdom" is made unconscious and unavailable.

Bollas (1987, 1992) writes of *existential memory* and of the *unthought known*. By existential memory, he alludes to the connection that escapes representation, a memory registered in every being. He maintains that children internalise the "maternal idiom" of care, which would be a complex way of being and of relating.

In his book *The Infinite Question* (2009), Bollas maintains that the communicative potential of the unconscious has been neglected in the analytic tradition in favour of the repressed unconscious: "We can see that all theoretical schools adopted Freud's theory of repression and dropped his theory of reception" (Bollas, 2009, p. 16). And again, "In effect, the theory of repression—allowed to occupy sole place within the history of psychoanalysis as the theory of unconscious—eliminated unconscious perception, unconscious organisation and unconscious communication from psychoanalytic theory" (Bollas, 2009, p. 16).

Starting from this point of view, we can distinguish two systems of the unconscious: the *dynamic* and the *emotional–receptive* unconscious.

The former corresponds to what was discovered and described by Freud (1915e) and is the *repressed* unconscious; the latter is what Bion (1962, 1992) intuited, the object of study by contemporary psychoanalysis that concerns *what we are not aware of*.

So if, therefore, the emotional unconscious exists alongside the dynamic unconscious, Freud tells us what would happen when the system that "lies below" (which permits psychic life) functions: a personal dynamic unconscious, permeated by relational conflicts and wishes, can be processed only in this case.

The emotional–receptive unconscious would represent the necessary condition for the existence and functioning of the dynamic unconscious, with which it would continuously relate.

Unconscious awareness

To return to the dream described earlier, it is clear that in order to formulate the thought contained in it, the patient uses an unconscious that has eyes to see. This unaware perception testifies to the capacity to correctly grasp one's own mental state and that of others through the emotional unconscious. Even though apparently under much suffering, some patients have a highly developed unconscious receptiveness that must be used and valued during the analytic process.

Preverbal emotional communication

Among many contemporary contributions, I mention only the work of Beebe and colleagues (1997). These authors attempt to cast some light on the early interactive structures that originate from the ways mother and infant communicate emotionally during the first year of life, before the use of words is possible. Their reciprocal exchanges organise the experience and create patterns that the child learns to recognise, expect, and remember. Later, these dyadic experiences are going to constitute the unconscious organisational structures that are the foundation of the personality. The authors describe a "pre-reflective", rather than a dynamic, unconscious; they also believe that the newborn's representations will be transcribed above all in the system of non-verbal representation.

These observations can be connected with Schore's (2003) assumptions related to neuroscientific data showing that non-verbal emotional communication between mother and infant (prosody, gestures, facial expressions), which is constantly occurring in the early months of care, allows for the formation of brain circuits situated in the orbital-frontal cortex and in the sub-cortical nuclei of the right hemisphere; this will be the biological support for the emotional unconscious life of the individual.

The consequent issue is that now we conceive the unconscious as not being given from the beginning, but, rather, as a system that develops progressively, if there are the necessary emotional conditions. This process is not always given and its lack has important consequences in terms of the individual's mental health.

Emotional receptors

The dynamic (repressed) unconscious and the emotional–receptive unconscious work in parallel. Before an emotion can be repressed, it needs to be captured and registered through a psychic receptor. In other words, the dynamic unconscious can perform its function of repressing the incompatible affect when this latter has been captured by the emotional receptors. First, the individual unknowingly registers the emotions, then he makes them unconscious if they feel incompatible.

Let me emphasise that repression can occur only when an emotion has been previously registered, in other words, if an unconscious exists that comes into action even before the dynamic unconscious.

However, things are not really as simple as this. It is not easy to describe how the emotional experiences are registered. Mostly, the repression process depends on the development of a receptive organ that can register emotions. According to my hypothesis, these conditions are missing in the more difficult (borderline and psychotic) patients.

What is unconscious for difficult patients?

My assumption is that at the root of the most severe pathologies there is a deterioration of the unconscious functions, in particular those upon which emotional awareness is based.

While neurosis results from a non-harmonious functioning of the dynamic unconscious, borderline or psychotic structures are nourished by an alteration of the emotional–receptive unconscious: that is, the mental apparatus capable of symbolising affects and using the emotional function of intrapsychic and relational communication.

Were we to compare the emotional–receptive unconscious with language, we would draw the conclusion that, in neuroses, the language that allows us to read the content is preserved; it is then a matter of articulating it better so that it becomes intelligible. In the case of borderline patients, we are confronted with a civilisation, the evolution of which towards language—that is, the possibility to structure and understand one's own history—could not be formed.

A similar distortion occurs in psychosis, where a communicative structure, such as the unconscious, is continually abused to build a solipsistic and grandiose world in which the receptive and communicative relational channels are obliterated.

Borderline pathology

In the clinical work with borderline patients, the conditions that we usually encounter with neurotic analysands are missing: both the transference as an expression of a conflict or an infantile wish and the capacity to dream—that is, to introduce emotional experiences in a narrative sequence, a form of attachment to the object with some constancy—are lacking.

Considering all the manifestations of the borderline symptomatology, for example, the fact that these patients oscillate continuously between moments of extreme dependence and moments of flight in their relationships as well as in the transference, we can think that, during their childhood and adolescence, the processes allowing for a development of symbolisation and a containment of the emotional states have never occurred (Garland, 2010).

The function of creating and maintaining relationships cannot take place and be represented in the form of memory, dream, narrative, or symbol. Rey (1994) describes borderline patients as persistently requesting things, as controllers, manipulators, intimidators, and belittlers. They blame society for their problems; they feel persecuted and might develop ideas of grandiosity. When they feel fragile, unprotected, and in danger, they may defend themselves with uncontrolled outbursts of rage and impulsive behaviour. These patients are dominated by violent emotions, but they are not able to describe or understand them, and certainly not process them.

In other words, the unconscious, as we are used to representing it, is not operating, not even in its function as a filter of repression. If consciousness is the capacity to register, memorise, and remember a psychic event, awareness concerns the meaning and understanding of that event. In these patients, awareness is the missing function.

Fonagy and Target (1996) postulate that patients with severe personality disorders inhibit a normal developmental stage of the mental processes (the reflective function), thus preventing understanding of the symbolic nuances of other people's behaviour. The problem highlighted on several occasions by Fonagy and his collaborators centres on the conditions that impede the structuring of the reflective faculties that would ensue from a missing maternal response to the infant's need for mirroring.

In the course of the analytic process with these patients, it is not sufficient to make the unconscious conscious; instead, it is important to develop the intuitive faculties that were originally missing. However, the difficulty lies in the fact that these patients are not capable of using associative thinking that allows an intuitive understanding of psychic facts. This lack of associations typical of these patients is also evident in the dreams that seem all too clear to the observer, but lack all meaning for the dreamer.

Psychosis

The emotional–receptive unconscious can be likened to implicit knowledge, which functions as an indispensable procedural memory for relational and emotional experiences. In the case of patients destined to develop a psychosis, this acquisition is damaged from the very beginning and suffers further injury from the psychopathological structures, such as, for example, the delusions that develop during the course of the illness.

A patient bound to become psychotic has lived in a withdrawal dissociated from reality—the secret place in which the psychosis will be created—for a very long time, the beginning of which dates back to infancy. In such a withdrawal, the patient does not use the mind as an instrument that allows him to intuit and think, but rather as a sense organ that produces pleasure in a dissociated way. And so he creates a world made up of visual images and concrete fantasies and obliterates the emotional functions that allow him to understand psychic reality.

The mental operations occurring in withdrawal are not subject to the laws of normal psychic functioning; they can be neither repressed nor "dreamt" in order to be transformed into thoughts. This gives rise to specific problems for therapists. Generally the operations that occur in the withdrawal are not described to the analyst because the patient himself is unaware of their pathogenic power and fails to foresee the consequences, such as, for example, when the delusion erupts.

Using the mind as a sense organ generates pleasant and exciting mental states at first, but then, as the process gets out of the patient's control, it creates distorted and anxiety-provoking perceptions, such as hallucinations that then torment him.

This very same kind of experience, which concerns a *sensory use* of the brain and where excitement replaces thinking, is also present in borderline patients to a lesser extent. In both types of patient, the manipulation of the perceptive organs reaches such a level that the receptive and intuitive function of the mind deteriorates progressively. While the borderline patients oscillate, getting in and out of these mental states, the psychotic ones enter a path that often turns out to be one of no return.

The origin of the problems

It is helpful to keep in mind that all the emotional experiences before the development of language contribute to construct the precursors of an internal emotional idiom that characterises the development of the unconscious psychic experience.

These patients are not able to repress in order to understand, and they are forced to expel the uncomfortable states through action; their capacity to isolate themselves, to use their body as a source of stimuli, and to treat the world of grandiose fantasies as the real world lies at the basis of this way of functioning. Hence, the difficulties for the analyst, who expects to dialogue with them by trying to use and clarify unconscious communications, and who, for a long time, cannot make use of symbolic interpretations that presuppose a correspondence between manifest content and repressed content, between conscious and unconscious.

It is not by accident that these patients cannot use associative thinking. Since the emotional states cannot be thought and contained, these patients work by short-circuiting, through automatic and impulsive responses (borderline) or constructing a parallel world of fantasy and fleeing into dissociated mental constructions (psychosis).

My reflections attempt to understand where the complexities of the treatment of some patients, who can only be called *difficult*, derive from. These individuals are, indeed, truly difficult to reach: some of them cannot even manage to respect the temporal aspect of the setting, regularly arriving late for sessions; they fail to organise their time and have great difficulty in remembering what has happened in the course of treatment. In particular, they do not suit the implicit conditions of analysis that bases its way of working on the presence of an available receptiveness on the part of the analysand.

Fonagy's hypothesis concerning a deficit in *reflective functioning* is very helpful for understanding what faculties are missing in these difficult patients; his definition, though, would seem to limit the damage to this particular function, whereas it is clear that the disorder is much wider ranging and affects all emotional functioning.

In the preceding pages, I have attempted to show how the border-line and psychotic organisations, while having different psycho-pathological dynamics, converge in the deficient functioning of the emotional–receptive unconscious.

One of the aims of analytic treatment is to develop the functions that enable awareness of oneself and one's emotions. Hence, it is important to prepare a specific setting (and we know how often the countertransference is difficult to handle) that allows those kinds of experiences that the patient has never experienced and has never tried before to develop. In other words, it is necessary to help him construct a real identity through his relationship with a new object.

PART II

CHAPTER EIGHT

The pathology of sexuality

"The insight has dawned on me that masturbation is the one major habit, the 'primary addiction,' and it is only as a substitute and replacement for it that the other addictions—to alcohol, morphine, tobacco, and the like—come into existence"

(Letter from Freud to Fliess, December 22, 1897, in Masson, 1985, p. 287)

Perverse sexualities are the result of precocious deviations in child development that become structured as pathological organisations that obliterate the child's evolutionary potential. In order to understand the nature of the perversion, it is important that we use the concept of *sexualisation* rather than that of sexuality. This distinction implies the existence of different categories of sexual experiences involving mental states that have little to do with ordinary sexuality.

Since the early days of psychoanalysis, sexuality has been awarded a central position in the psychoanalytic discipline, so much so that the term was used to denote Freud's psychosexual theory; however, with the affirmation of the theory of object relations, it has been transformed into a secondary effect of the affective relational bond. This is why I believe it is useful to describe the role assigned to sexuality in the various theoretical models and to differentiate *sexuality in clinical work* from *sexuality in theory*, with a special focus on pathological sexuality.

In my view, a pathological distortion of the sexual sphere is already present in the infancy of those individuals who go on to develop a sexual disorder in adulthood.

I hope these preliminary remarks will help to trigger a useful discussion that will aid our understanding of the genesis, evolution, and therapy of the more serious distortions of sexuality, such as, for example, the perversions.

Is theory being desexualised?

For several years now, a lively debate about sexuality has been engaging the international psychoanalytic community. Green (1997) was the first to raise the issue, postulating that post-Freudian theoretical and clinical models had *desexualised* psychoanalytic thought. In fact, the Freudian interpretative model, which explains mental illness as an arrest or distortion of the development of the libido (in Freud, psyche and soma are intimately interwoven), is disappearing from analytic papers and publications.

According to the French analyst, the observations deriving from infant research, the conceptualisation of object relations, and the study of borderline patients have overshadowed the significance of sexuality in psychoanalysis; it is no longer considered a decisive factor in child development or a useful criterion for understanding clinical psychopathology. In Green's opinion, its diminished importance has impoverished psychoanalytic thought.

Green believes that Klein's theories about emotional development are largely responsible for this change: her object-relations theory would seem to preclude any opportunity for attributing the right level of importance to "the intrapsychic consequences of the sexual drives that do not readily lend themselves to observation [and that] prove to be minimised in the resulting theoretical reformulation" (Green, 1997, p. 347).[10]

Green's reasoning undoubtedly serves to underline the fact that for some time a distinct divide had been widening between Freud's original hypothesis, which linked psychic development to sexual maturity, and subsequent psychoanalytic investigation that was leading in very different directions.

The discussion initiated by the French analyst also touched on the issue of the relationship between clinical work and theory. Is it only a theoretical shift that has weakened the notion of sexuality in psychoanalysis, or does a divergence really exist between the psychosexual model and true sexuality?

On this point, Stein (1998) points out that the theme of the International Psychoanalytical Association (IPA) Congress in Barcelona (1997), "Psychoanalysis and Sexuality", in which the term "sexuality" replaced that of "psychosexuality", implied that psychoanalysis could be separated from sexuality, a phenomenon that invites reflection. Fonagy (2006), too, adds that the title was very significant, since the main psychoanalytic theories had developed from bases other than that of sexuality, and goes on to confirm that in the psychoanalytic literature of recent decades there has been a progressive disappearance of the term "sexuality" and its correlates.

Psychosexuality

On a number of occasions, Freud stated that the search for pleasure is a characteristic of man that is manifest from the earliest stages of life; even the baby seeks and experiences pleasure, whereas sexuality is fundamental because it stimulates and organises the development of psychic life.

Sexuality is the determining element of the psychosexual theory because it has an aim and an object; its phases can be described and represented in quantitative terms. Furthermore, it also allows the various psychopathological syndromes to be classified in a hierarchical order, from the most serious—those fixed at the earliest levels of development—to the less serious of the later phases.

While considering sexuality in a positive light, Freud did not undervalue its pathogenic power; in a letter of 22 December 1897 to his friend and colleague, Fliess, he affirms that masturbation is the first drug known to man. These are his words:

> The insight has dawned on me that masturbation is the one major habit, the "primary addiction," and it is only as a substitute and replacement for it that the other addictions—to alcohol, morphine, tobacco, and the like—come into existence. (Masson, 1985, p. 287)

In a very schematic way, three successive periods can be observed in Freud's thought that correspond to three theoretical points of view about sexuality.

In the first period, which concludes with *Studies on Hysteria* (1895d), Freud identifies the pathogenic agent of neurosis in sexuality, which he theorises as the traumatic aetiology (later modified). The *sexuality* he refers to is that of *conventional* language, of repressed sexual and loving desire.

In the second period, Freud advances a general theory of the individual's development that is founded on psychosexuality, with the libido an expression of the drive. In the libido theory, and in keeping with the pre-eminence of the pleasure principle, the notion of sexuality broadens to include every form of bodily pleasure. All sensory forms of pleasure are primitive components of the libido: even the baby's sensory pleasure in sucking is an expression of sexuality. In this instinctual model, sexuality is considered to be a unitary process: the quantitative difference, the level of arousal, would explain the different psychopathological outcomes.

The third period coincides with the turning point that occurred in 1920 (Freud, 1920g): sexuality, contrasted with the death instinct, now corresponds to the positive force of love that counters the destructiveness that tends to pull apart and divide. Sexuality is no longer a primitive aggressive force, a partial perverse–polymorphous instinct, but Eros in constant struggle with Thanatos.

It might be said, therefore, that the *desexualising* process of psychoanalysis was initiated by Freud himself. After theorising the death instinct (1920g), he modified his conception of the meaning and role of sexuality in mental life. However, it was not a complete break, but a continuous process that developed through a succession of models that accompanied the evolution of Freud's thought.

The analysts that followed him (for example, Klein, Bion, and Winnicott) attributed greater importance to the relational and emotional aspects of development. In fact, the sexual experience of the child is not denied, but it is no longer considered to be so important for development.

In conclusion, if sexuality has lost its original importance in analytic theory, this is due to a shift in the interpretative paradigms of child development and to the introduction of theoretical parameters that differ from the original one. Theoretical change has enabled the successful assertion of a number of different concepts in which sexuality has given way to other important factors of development.

Finally, it is necessary to distinguish the theoretical level, whose parameters have altered, from the clinical one: in the latter, in fact, one frequently comes across erotic and sexual experiences of a pathological nature (sexualised transference and withdrawals, perverse fantasies, and so on) that must be understood in their multi-form meaning.

Sensoriality and sexuality

During the progressive transformation of Freud's theory, sexuality was always conceived as a unitary force: its expressions vary; it has aggressive or gentle components, it can bind with and oppose the destructive instinct, but it remains within a unitary model. Freud conceives sexuality as a unitary process, even though he describes the different phases of psychosexual development and the shift in the libido organisation (oral, anal, phallic). Similarly, every sensory aspect forms with a part of the pleasure of sexuality. However, this formulation gives rise to certain issues: for example, the theoretical equivalence between *sensoriality* and *sexuality*.

I would like to quote an entire passage from *Three Essays on the Theory of Sexuality* (Freud, 1905d) to better clarify Freud's thought process:

> A child's intercourse with anyone responsible for his care affords him an unending source of sexual excitation and satisfaction from his erotogenic zones. This is especially so since the person in charge of him, who, after all, is as a rule his mother, herself regards him with feelings that are derived from her own sexual life: she strokes him, kisses him, rocks him and quite clearly treats him as a substitute for a complete sexual object. A mother would probably be horrified if she were made aware that all her marks of affection were rousing her child's sexual instinct and preparing for its later intensity. She regards what she does as asexual, "pure" love, since, after all, she carefully

avoids applying more excitations to the child's genitals than are unavoidable in nursery care. As we know, however, the sexual instinct is not aroused only by direct excitation of the genital zone. What we call affection will unfailingly show its effects one day on the genital zones as well. Moreover, if the mother understood more of the high importance of the part played by instincts in mental life as a whole – in all its ethical and psychical achievements – she would spare herself any self-reproaches even after her enlightenment. She is only fulfilling her task in teaching the child to love ... It is true that an excess of parental affection does harm by causing precocious sexual maturity ... And on the other hand neuropathic parents, who are inclined as a § rule to display excessive affection, are precisely those who are most likely by their caresses to arouse the child's disposition to neurotic illness. (Freud, 1905d, p. 223)

Two directions of intimately connected but potentially divergent reasoning emerge in this excerpt. The first regards the development of normal sexuality. Freud senses that the mother's loving warmth is necessary for the child's emotional growth as this will enable him to enjoy good sexuality as an adult; at the same time, it points to the risk of adult sexuality intruding into the child's mind. When the mother uses her child for purposes of arousal (neuropathic parents), the latter's sexuality may easily develop precociously. In this case, the parent does not perceive the child's need for affection, but projects into him his/her own eroticised excitement.

The implicit link is to Ferenczi's "Confusion of tongues between adults and the child", which will be written much later (1933). Here, Freud also anticipates Khan's (1963) conceptualisation of cumulative trauma, in which an excess of erotic stimulation on the part of the parent sets the child on the path towards perversion.

The complex nature of the passage derives from the fact that Freud merges both *sensoriality* and *sexuality* in his concept of sexuality. By not differentiating between the two, he runs the risk of standardising moments that have a different significance from the *emotional point of view*. Even if caresses are a preliminary pleasure that precedes the practice of adult sexuality, they are also a means for exchanging affection outside a sexual context.

Conceptualising sexuality as a unitary factor led Freud to conceive adult perversions as resulting from a lack of inhibition of infantile sexuality. Already, in his letter of 6 December 1896 to Fliess, he noted,

"For another consequence of premature sexual experiences is perversion, of which the determinant seems to be that defence either does not occur before the psychic apparatus is completed or does not occur at all" (Masson, 1985, p. 210).

The psychosexual model, formulated later, would allow Freud to place all the perversions in the spheres of the sexual drive.

Development without sexuality

Balint (1956) lists two possible ways for classifying perversion. The first, which refers to the Freudian theory of partial instincts and to the different organisations of the libido, links the perversion to infantile forms of sexuality. But this definition runs aground with both homosexuality (if that is considered a perversion) and with sadomasochism (which is difficult to consider as an infantile form of psychosexual development).

The second, based on the relational theory, underlines the difference between genital love and perversion, specifying that, in the latter, a form of love for a human object is missing.

Klein introduced a new way of conceiving child sexuality, claiming that psycho-emotional development follows a different path from sexuality. The processes of introjection and identification, both necessary to growth, take place without implying sexual fantasying. While Freud maintained that sexuality organises the psyche, Klein believes that the psyche organises the type of sexuality. The child of Kleinian theory is moved by love and by hate; the prevalence of one of the two positions will be decisive for the direction his sexuality takes. In particular, Klein maintains that when the level of anxiety in the child is too high, the arrival of sexuality does not represent real development but, instead, a defence, a flight from an excess of anxiety.

This idea opened the way for identifying normal sexual development from a *flight into sexuality*, in other words, a non-relational and self-stimulating practice.

Inherent problems in the unitary model

The assumption that adult sexual disorder is nothing but an accentuation of some aspects of infantile sexuality is also present in the theories of analysts who have contributed in an original way to the problem of sexuality and who do not adhere completely to the psychosexual model.

Kernberg (1995) holds that every sexual gratification contains unconscious fantasies with sadistic, masochistic, exhibitionist, and voyeuristic elements. Sadomasochism is not just a pathology limited to perverse subjects, but an essential component of sexual fantasy in general; indeed, Kernberg believes that when it reaches a heightened level, sexual arousal verges on the fantasy world of perversion and pornography.

In linking together erotic arousal and perversion, other analysts (Chodorow, 1992; McDougall, 1995) believe that, at least in fantasy, there is little difference between normal sexuality and perversion. For example, McDougall (1995) explains the blend between normality and perversion with the ever-present pre-genital urges and organisation of the primitive internal objects.

In other words, these models take their origin from Freud's hypotheses, which, in starting from the monism of psychosexuality, make no distinction between perversion and infantile polymorphous sexuality.

I believe that perversion draws on sexuality but, unlike infantile polymorphism, it contains a pathological component that differs totally from the child's normal search for sensory pleasure. In this sense, I feel very close to Meltzer (1973), who clearly differentiates *polymorphous* from *perverse* and *immature sexuality*.

The distinction between primitive and pathological is particularly important when trying to place the problematic issues of sexual disorders in the right perspective.

As Fonagy (2005) notes, in psychoanalysis there is an unjustified trust in the possibility of associating some particular psychopathologies to specific stages of development. Freud himself conceived illness as a quantitatively anomalous development of structures and physiological functionings active in the earliest phases of an individual's growth.

An example of the equivalence between primitive and pathological is given by the infantile sexuality present, according to Freud, in many neurotic mental processes and in particular, as claimed by the psychosexual model, in perversion.

Even Klein followed the same principle: in her infant therapies, she maintained that sadism, present in the fantasies that the child communicates in the consulting room, derives from the sadistic–anal stage of physiological development.

In contrast to the view that sees the primitive coinciding with the pathological, no evidence demonstrates that the adult disorder is a repetition of a normal child development; on the contrary, various studies have shown that illness in adults is preceded by evident infant disorders in 75% of cases (Kim-Cohen et al., 2003).

A very important contribution to this theme comes from Caper (1998), who questioned the equivalence between the primitive and the pathological, making a clear distinction between the two terms. He wonders whether the adult illness can be conceived as a fixation or a regression to a primitive mental state, by this intending a precocious stage of normal psychological development, or whether a clear difference exists between normal and pathological development.

He postulates that the sick adult is the result of an already sick child and that it is incorrect to maintain that the psychopathology is a regression or a fixation to a normal primitive stage because, in doing so, one runs the risk of confusing, from a theoretical and clinical point of view, the destructive phases of the mind with normal and primitive ones capable of development.

Three paradigms

As a whole, the psychoanalytic theories that deal with sexual disorders can be divided into three basic groups.[11]

In the first, the theories are based on the psychosexual model, faithful to Freud's ideas, and consider sexual disorders as the crystallisation of libidinal and aggressive tendencies that characterise the evolution of human sexuality. The contribution of Chasseguet-Smirgel (1985) is the most modern and coherent version of this theoretical approach.

In the second group, relational theories place the emphasis on the defensive function of sexuality, considering the anxieties that threaten personal identity to be fundamental for understanding the perversion. Authors following this trend adhere to the ideas of Winnicott and others, such as the North American analysts, who follow in the steps of Kohut. For the latter, perversion is a narcissistic object relation potentially directed towards more integrated forms of the Self's structuring.

Third, other currents of Kleinian inspiration consider perversion, which becomes structured as a psychopathological organisation of the personality, as a sexualisation of power and cruelty. Sexuality, the expression of the internal world, can be considered perverse only when components interested in power and in belittling the object prevail.

Child sexuality and orgasmic pleasure

In his paper "'A child is being beaten'", Freud (1919e) describes a number of young patients who, at a very early age (four or five years), reach orgasm by identifying with the person hitting the child or with the hit child. In other words, these children, still very young and on the basis of sadomasochistic fantasies, reach orgasm, a mental state normally precluded from the infantile experience.

The presence or not of orgasm in the child should help to distinguish between normal and pathological "child sexuality", between *sensoriality* and *sexualisation*.

Characterised by bodily pleasure, child sexuality should not arrive at orgasm, which is possible only when the sexual organs have matured. The normal child's pleasure is limited to the *sensory sphere*, where a part of the body or its orifices are used to produce infantile sensory pleasure, which, moreover, persists into adult life in preparation for sexual enjoyment, which will reach its peak in orgasm.

How do these children reach orgasm if it is normally reached only after the genitals have biologically matured and they are manipulated? Are we in the presence of sexuality, or of sexualised processes of the mind?

The fact is that these children reach orgasmic pleasure without genital manipulation and only through arousal produced by fantasies (in this case of a sadistic or masochistic nature).

It is also possible for adults to reach orgasm without any bodily stimulation. Komisaruk and colleagues (2006) have shown in the laboratory that some individuals can reach orgasm only by using the imagination, with no bodily stimulation whatsoever. These people are capable of doing something awake that normally occurs while dreaming, when the dreamer ejaculates during an erotic dream. The data collected in the laboratory show that during orgasm obtained with the imagination, the same areas of the brain are activated that come into play during orgasm reached by genital stimulation.

This helps us to understand why some children are capable of experiencing orgasm even when sexually immature: they reach it through the power of fantasying because they have *sexualised* psychic reality. In this case, *adult (orgasmic) sexuality* has penetrated the infant life and, from this moment onwards, will determine its development (and psychopathology). When adults, these children will not be capable of experiencing relational sexuality and will remain arrested within a withdrawal of perverse arousal.

The distinction between *child sensoriality, sexuality,* and *sexualisation processes* is extremely important in our clinical work for understanding the dynamics of sexual disorders and perversions; infantile sexualisation processes are the precise elements on which the nucleus of the perverse structures is established.

This significant differentiation has a bearing on the entire clinical scheme of the following three chapters. The basic idea underlying all of them is that perversion does not correspond to the development of infantile polymorphous sexuality, but is a flight and a withdrawal that begins in infancy with the production of sexualised mental states; the deprived child easily discovers masturbatory mental states and uses his body to support and defend himself from depressive falls.

CHAPTER NINE

The erotic transference:
from dream to delusion*

"We believe that love will solve all problems, when love is the prize for having solved all problems"

(Anonymous)

T
he erotic transference can be thought of as the two-faced Janus of analytical clinical work: it can be triggered by positive emotions that are necessary for building new shared realities or draw its nourishment from distorted, falsified constructions. In the former case, the erotic transference expresses the capacity to antici-pate, to "dream" the emotional relationship with the object and this is why Freud valued its transformative aspect as a driving force towards change. In contrast, in the latter it amounts to a flight from psychic reality and can be transformed into a real delusion.

This chapter seeks to illustrate the various clinical forms of the erotic transference and the different ways of treating them. It is no

* This paper was first presented at the International Psychoanalytical Association Congress in Chicago, 21 December 2009. Translated by Philip Slotkin, MA, Cantab. MITI.

simple matter to distinguish between the mental states that emerge in the course of the erotic transference, and neither is it easy to tell them apart from other analytic phenomena, since this type of transference seems to be not so much an isolated clinical fact as, in effect, a frontier region contiguous with many kinds of clinical experience. The erotic transference is observed in a number of psychopathological syndromes, such as the neuroses (in particular, hysteria), depression, borderline states, and even psychosis.

Two types of clinical situation can be distinguished. The first corresponds to an analysable transference potentially capable of transformation, and resembles a state of dreaming reminiscent of an ideal infantile love. The second, which is malignant in nature and appears similar to a drugged or delusional state, proves much more difficult to treat. I shall present some clinical examples to demonstrate the differences and possible therapeutic approaches.

Freud and transference love

The notion of erotic transference is very old-established, in fact dating back to the earliest days of psychoanalysis: the history of our discipline (Jones, 1953) indicates that the main reason for the split between Freud and Breuer was the latter's inability to withstand the erotic transference of Anna O.[12] Psychoanalysis, according to this version, has paradoxical origins, the erotic transference having caused one of its two pioneers to abandon it.

A partial explanation of the significance of the erotic transference was given by Freud in 1914, who discusses it systematically in "Observations on transference-love", emphasising that no doctor who experiences it "will find it easy to retain his grasp on the analytic situation and to keep clear of the illusion that the treatment is really at an end" (Freud, 1915a, p. 162). He adds that the phenomenon is one of the "particular expressions of resistance", and, in particular, that the patient seeks "to destroy the doctor's authority by bringing him down to the level of a lover" (p. 163).

In other words, Freud is clearly stating that the erotic transference is an attempt by the patient to escape from what would later be called the dependent infantile transference ("destroy[ing] the doctor's authority"). However, this analytic situation is not merely an expression of resistance, but, in fact, contains the potential for development. Freud writes (1915a, p. 165) that

> . . . the patient's need and longing should be allowed to persist in her, in order that they may serve as forces impelling her to do work and to make changes, and that we must beware of appeasing those forces by means of surrogates

by suggesting, for instance, that the offers of love be set aside, or, on the other hand, that they be accepted, even if only platonically.

If nothing else, it is clear that the analyst must avoid ending up like the pastor in Freud's famous anecdote, who hurries to the bedside of a dying insurance agent to convert him, but leaves with an insurance policy while the agent remains true to his convictions.

What matters for Freud, therefore, is to keep the erotic transference alive so that its roots in infancy can be uncovered. He recommends treating the patient's love as something *unreal*, which, he adds, is not easy in the case of certain women who are "accessible only to 'the logic of soup, with dumplings for arguments'", who "tolerate no surrogates": with "such people one has the choice between returning their love or else bringing down upon oneself the full enmity of a woman scorned" (1915a, pp. 166–167).

Caught as he is between Scylla and Charybdis—between gratification and frustration—the analyst must put his trust in his analytic skills if he is not to be seduced by the patient's Sirens (Hill, 1994, p. 485).

What is *unreal* for Freud is that this love is a virtually stereotypic repetition of the patient's experience of his past and of his infancy; while this love is not ultimately directed to the analyst, what love, one wonders, is not, in fact, a repetition of the past?

At the end of this paper, Freud enquires whether the love for the analyst can indeed be deemed unreal, and, respectful of the extraordinary nature of this analytic phenomenon, suspends his investigation at this point.

Freud hesitates between the alternatives of the loving transference as a defence against the relationship of dependence and as real love. Is this transference a compulsion to repeat the past, a defence against the new, or, on the other hand, a potent analytic bond, a force "impelling [the patient] to . . . make changes": that is, to embrace the new?

The reality of the new relationship is confirmed by the observation that interpretations intended to take the patient back to the past often merely wound him just when he is relinquishing his age-old defences against affectionate experiences and turning with passion towards the analyst.

A historical interlude

By way of introduction, I should like to recall a well-known event from the history of psychoanalysis. The year 1977 saw the discovery in the vaults of Geneva's Palais Wilson of a box of private documents, including the diary of Sabina Spielrein and the Freud–Jung correspondence. Some of these documents were published in an interesting volume edited by Aldo Carotenuto (1982), who was the first to reveal the story of the love between Sabina and Jung.[13]

In 1904, Sabina Spielrein, not yet eighteen years old, was admitted to the Burghölzli psychiatric clinic in Zurich for symptoms diagnosed as a hysterical psychosis or crisis of schizophrenia. Here, she underwent two months of analytic treatment with Jung, who used a technique that, while admittedly of its time (associations and abreaction of the traumatic infantile complex), was underpinned by the passion of the pioneer and the generosity of the man. The fact is that Sabina soon left the hospital and enrolled at the university to study medicine. Jung encouraged her and, as her therapy continued, allowed the relationship to become increasingly intimate, with a growing admixture of mutual idealisation. In her sessions, Jung came to represent such a model of heroism that, in Sabina's fantasy, he assumed the name of Siegfried, Wagner's mythical hero. In the diary discovered in Geneva, Sabina describes in detail the atmosphere of passion and of mystical union with the figure of her hero. Thus, there developed a passionate transference of enormous proportions that endowed her with intense vitality and foreshadowed a grandiose destiny for both protagonists.

Jung set the young Sabina aflame by confessing to her that he had similar thoughts to hers. This strongly suggests that she was able to read the mind of her analyst-cum-friend and could sense through premonitory dreams that he, too, wished to have a child with her. Jung, however, swung between an idealised declaration of his own love and the attempt to damp down an awkward relationship whose outcome was unforeseeable.

The diary reveals the young patient's stubborn and relentless endeavours to make her analyst understand the nature and significance of the passionate fantasy that impelled her towards him. The dream of uniting with the hero was a mystical disposition that underlay Sabina's creativity, just as she was composing some personal essays in which she engaged in a dialogue with Jung, thus—at the age of barely twenty-one—foreshadowing some of the themes that she was to develop later in her scientific contributions. Jung, who had previously poured fuel on these fantasies, now sought to reduce their intensity by interpretation; Sabina, on the other hand, fought with all her might against him and against his attempt to withdraw and to ascribe everything to the vicissitudes of the libido.

Sabina remained prominent in the circle of Freud's pupils, and was even dispatched to teach psychoanalysis at the Rousseau Institute in Geneva, where one of her training analysands was to be the young Piaget.

The erotico–passionate transference to Jung, unanalysed and untransformed, was not extinguished and stayed with Sabina Spielrein over the years. In some of the surviving letters to Jung, Sabina, now married and pregnant with her second child, complained that "Siegfried", the son she had had in fantasy by Jung, might resurface as an inner presence likely to interfere with the forthcoming birth.

Some analytic contributions

Blum (1973) describes the various possible configurations of the erotic transference, ranging from relatively minor forms with positive and affectionate aspects to the extreme cases he defines as erotised transferences, accompanied by explicit offers of sex.

Blum takes issue with Rappaport's (1959) view that the erotic transference always involves a deficiency of reality testing or an ego disturbance typical of borderline and psychotic patients; he contends that progress in therapy depends not on the manifest symptoms, but on the patient's capacity for development.

Another important contribution to the subject was made by Schafer (1977), who examines the reality or unreality of the loving transference and concludes that transference love is equivalent to a kind of transitional state, at one and the same time real and unreal, progressive and regressive, whereby the patient attempts to reconcile fantasy with reality and an old attitude with a possible new one. Schafer points out that every transference involves multiple realities and meanings, and that this is particularly true of the erotic transference.

Examining the nature of the "love" and "sexuality" encountered in the loving transference, I (De Masi, 1988) would like to emphasise the discontinuity between idealisation, erotisation, and sexualisation that characterises different forms of erotic transference with contrasting clinical outcomes.

Bolognini (1994), too, considers the erotic transference, which he subdivides into four types, erotised, erotic, loving, and affectionate, the first being accompanied by psychotic and the second by neurotic functioning. Loving and affectionate transferences constitute clinical forms resembling healthy development, differing from each other according to the level of maturation of the Oedipus complex.

With these contributions in mind, I shall attempt in this chapter to explain the meaning of the erotic transference in the various mental states, with particular attention to the presence or absence of the sexual component proper. I shall call the forms that lack actual sexual elements *loving* or *idealising transferences*, reserving the epithet *erotic* or *sexualised* for the type of transference in which the wish is specifically sexual. I shall also consider the "unreality" of this transference, which alternates between the "dream" of love and actual delusion.

Idealisation in the loving transference

Madeleine, about thirty years old and of French origin, has come into analysis because the suffering she has experienced since adolescence has worsened over the years. She lives alone, concentrating on her career, from which she derives little pleasure. Her family, which includes two older brothers, has remained in France. Madeleine does not suffer from loneliness, and has not aspired to a love relationship, since the ones she embarked on in the past all came to nothing.

In the first part of Madeleine's analysis, dreams of marshes and constricted spaces from which she would like to emerge seem to express a wish to escape from the isolation in which she has been confined for many years.

For a long time, it is hard to identify an emotional bond with myself. For example, my attempts to discern in her any form of disturbance in anticipation of analytic separations are met with scepticism and incredulity.

I am both surprised and caught off guard when, after several sessions in which she told me about the towns, perfumes, and casbahs of Morocco, she announces that she has fallen in love with me, adding that she would like to travel with me to these places. In my attempt to put her declaration of love in perspective, I evince some manifest embarrassment, as the patient does not mention the subject again; moreover, she tells me in the next session that on the previous evening she almost yielded to the sexual advances of a man she had met at the home of some friends. In the ensuing sessions, too, she behaves as if the declaration of love had never been made.

I am convinced that it is important to take up this matter again and, after a few weeks, I try to work with her to understand the reason for the silence that followed her declaration. Madeleine tells me that she was hurt by my response to her profession of love, and therefore blotted out any feelings connected with it. Her attraction to me was like a dream that had faded away when I was unwilling to share in it. As we discuss the situation, it becomes clear that the loving transference is not oedipal in character, but has to do with the aspiration to be one with the mother, in contact with the sensory beauty of nature. This must have represented the primal deficiency in her infancy that impelled her to engage in a privileged relationship with her father during her adolescence, when she even shared with him the experience of work and leisure.

As the analysis progresses, it gradually becomes possible to consider in depth the various aspects of the experience of the loving transference.

Madeleine explains that an important component of the dream of love was the wish for oneness with me: we would have travelled together, and she would have been able to see the world through my eyes. Now she realises how much she, instead, aspires to achieve a separate identity of her own and to experience things at first hand. She does not deny that her declaration was also that of a woman in search of a love relationship, but feels that the dreaming aspect was predominant and that she expected me to respond in kind. My response had hurt her, and she had therefore withdrawn. Yet, she thinks it important to have been able to experience such a passionate state of mind for the first time in her life.

At an advanced stage in her analysis, the patient says that she no longer feels that she is in love with me as in that episode from the past; she is fond of me, respects me, and is grateful to me for the experience of analysis, but is keenly aware of the differences that separate us, so she cannot see me as similar to her or share her life with me in the same way. Madeleine has, in effect, for the first time, become able to perceive the difference between generations; now she can see me as a parent figure, unlike her experience of her father, with whom she had a relationship that was both privileged and confused.

* * *

A particularity of this patient's loving transference is the absence of a sexual component; she herself claims not be censoring erotic fantasies about me—she simply does not have any. In the past, this woman had sexual experiences without emotional involvement. Examination of the sequence—the declaration of love in the session followed by sexual acting out in the outside world—clearly shows that the acting out was a defensive manoeuvre directed against the declaration (and against my unempathic response), which had left her too exposed. However, the dream of love experienced for the first time in the analysis seems to be an initial attempt to achieve at last the emotional involvement necessary for the genuine passionate cathexis of a love object.

As to my countertransference position, I must say that the patient's declaration at first seemed to be that of an adult woman to an adult man, hence my assumption that it contained an erotic offer. In other words, I took the patient's communication at face value and even briefly commented that the cultivation of a love relationship appeared inconsistent with her need to develop an analytic relationship. This misapprehension on my part was, I believe, the disturbing factor that caused the patient to feel that she had not been understood and to distance herself from the situation. I now think that my response to the patient's declaration of love was an example of Ferenczi's (1955[1933]) "confusion of tongues". It became clear from our subsequent exchanges that she had spoken the language of a child expressing its love for its mother, while I had been unable to understand and to respond empathically because I was influenced by the adult vision of love, which includes an erotic component.

Whereas the prospect of going on a trip together had appeared to me to be at variance with analysis, for the patient it represented a primary experience of contact with the mother's mind, and, hence, consistent with her analytic development. Some time before, the patient had had a dream in which my wife invited her to go out and explore the world around her, which ought to have enlightened me as to the nature of her declaration of "love". Hence the absence of a sexual correlate, because what was involved was, in fact, a primal, ideal relationship with a mother figure that had been lacking in her experience. By not responding to her on the right level, I had compelled her to attempt to move on while leaving this important step in maturation unresolved. The type of loving transference I am describing here corresponds to a painful state of emotional exaltation that mixes object loss with the possibility of ideal union with the object. Precisely because such an absolute demand is the expression of a heightened return to primal needs, it is perhaps most likely to be exhibited by patients whose earliest experiences of dependence underwent traumatic interference.

This compound of affection and longing is encountered in some patients who, at difficult times such as analytic separations, remain attached to their analysis, fantasising the gentle, ideal, and continuous presence of the analyst; a precarious balance arises in the analysis between an idealised state and an ongoing underlying sense of loss.

I postulate that such idealising loving transferences are benign in character and convey the essence of emotional experiences that were suppressed in infancy, perhaps owing to a lack of receptivity in the primal object (the mother). These emotions will resurface in analysis when the appropriate conditions for an affective relationship with the analyst are established. This type of transference, characterised as it is by longing and melancholic feelings, is, in part, an attempt to compensate for the pain of loss during analytic separations; however, it is also an expression of that pain.

When the analyst becomes a permanent figure in the patient's internal world, the experience of presence and of loss can be worked through and can become the prototype of a good emotional relationship.

The idealised loving transference is pre-oedipal in nature and exists independently of differences in gender; it can develop in both male and female patients. It is indicative of a relationship of longing with a mother who was present at the dawn of growth but suddenly disappeared from the infant's life, thus compelling the infant to distance himself from the world of emotional relationships.

A parallel reality

Some of the analysts who have addressed the subject of the erotic transference (Gould, 1994; Person, 1985; Rappaport, 1959) have rightly pointed out that this mental state involves a loss of contact with reality. In the erotic transference, regarded as a repetition of the relationship with the mother or father of infancy, the analyst forfeits his role as a bridge to the past and becomes the object of erotic desire.

I should now like to consider the problem in terms of the relationship between, first, withdrawal into fantasy and, second, psychic reality.

Winnicott (1971, p. 26) draws an important distinction between dreaming and psychic reality, on the one hand, and fantasying, on the other. In his view, dreaming has to do with emotional reality: "Dream fits into object-relating in the real world, and living in the real world fits into the dream-world . . .". Conversely, "fantasying remains an isolated phenomenon, absorbing energy but not contributing-in either to dreaming or to living".

Dreams and real-life experiences can be repressed, whereas fantasies have a different fate: "Inaccessibility of fantasying is associated with dissociation rather than with repression" (Winnicott, 1971, p. 27). Winnicott points out in a footnote (1971, p. 30) that this mental state of omnipotence must be distinguished from the "experience of omnipotence", which has to do with the alternate experiencing of "me" and "not-me". The latter experience belongs to dependence, while the former has its origins in hopelessness about dependence.

In other words, Winnicott is drawing attention to the need to distinguish between the world of fantasy and creative imagination, on the one hand, and *withdrawal into fantasy*, as some patients do, on the other. It does indeed seem that some patients value a life of withdrawal into fantasy more than the possibility of experiencing the reality of human relations. The existence of this fantasy world is the reason for the loss of reality that characterises the erotic transference: the withdrawal into fantasy is counterposed with, and replaces, psychic reality. These two realities coexist for long periods without ever meeting.

This situation is illustrated by the following case history from a recent supervision.

* * *

After a difficult childhood, Fausta soon left home and married a man of her own age. However, it quickly became evident that he was unsuited to married life, having confessed to her that he was a homosexual, thus triggering a crisis in the patient's life, as a result of which she came into analysis apparently suffering from severe depression.

Although the analysis was seemingly going well and the patient was benefiting from it, the analyst was becoming increasingly aware of an intense idealisation of himself. He often appeared in her dreams as a guide or as someone intent on engaging in intimate affective exchanges with her. The idealisation of the analyst was paralleled by the disparagement of her current partner (she always chose partners whose characters left much to be desired and who readily lent themselves to disparagement).

The analyst had tried many times, perhaps without sufficient conviction, to draw the patient's attention to this excessively idealised relationship, but although she seemed to accept what he said, it had had no effect.

The erotic transference found overt expression towards the fourth year in a drama that followed an exchange at the end of a session. As the patient was paying her fee for the month, the analyst noticed that only his first name was written on the envelope containing the money. In response to his questioning posture, she explained that this was a way of making the therapist anonymous: only the analyst's first name and not his surname appeared in her diary, too. The analyst remarked that it also seemed to be a representation of a secret relationship; his comment was intentional, with the aim of encouraging the patient to confront the issue in her sessions. Next time, however, the patient failed to mention it, and instead talked about her problems at work.

She began the next-but-one session by bringing a dream:

"Last night you and I had sex for the first time. I've never dreamt that we were having sex, but at most that you were giving me a kiss. You were very gentle and sensitive, and I enjoyed that a lot. You were touching my nipples and I was having oral sex with you. I particularly noticed that you seemed to be enjoying it, but in such a way that I didn't know if it was genuine or if you were exaggerating."

The patient herself associated the dream to the exchange that hinted at a possible secret relationship. She said she very much liked it when her nipples were touched, and repeated that the analyst/partner's pleasure in the dream was very intense, almost as if he was in part putting on an act. She commented that she could now talk to him about these things relatively calmly, whereas in the past she would not have done so.

She then remembered the initial part of the dream before the erotic scene:

"I came to your house and you were married. One of the people there was your wife . . . I felt at ease, but I noticed that you were looking at me in a particular way, as if you were winking at me . . . Then the atmosphere changed and it all happened . . . That surprised me, because although you hadn't had any erotic experience with me, you seemed to know how to pleasure me, and I knew how to do it for you too . . . but it wasn't really a sexual relationship; it was something else . . ."

*   *   *

Although the erotic dream was partly inspired by the exchange at the end of the session when she paid her fee, the analyst's remark had triggered the parallel reality that had been cultivated by the patient for a long time: a fleeting, suggestive exchange of glances had sufficed to plunge her into the erotic situation.

The dream is, in my view, important because it features both realities—the oedipal reality (given that the analyst's wife also appears in the first part of the dream) and the dissociated erotised reality. The patient demonstrates in the dream how easy it is to move back and forth between them.

A closer look at the erotic situation described in the dream indicates that the patient enjoys arousing the analyst, who, in turn, makes a point of showing off his arousal in order to heighten the patient's performance and to arouse her. By working on this aspect of the dream, the patient understood that she was unable to resist the fascination of arousing her partner, and that, therefore, she always ended up choosing easily seducible partners.

She accepted the analyst's interpretation and acknowledged her tendency—projected in the dream on to the analyst—to fake a pleasure that sometimes did not exist. She admitted that, in the analysis, too, she perhaps skipped over things that were not to her liking. In other words, it was becoming increasingly clear that remaining in a superficial relationship without ever making genuine contact was a speciality of this patient, who had never in her life allowed herself to experience a genuine love relationship.

Love, for her, consisted not so much in the wish to relate to a valued partner as in the ability to experience in fantasy something that aroused her. For this reason, she needed to find malleable men who were easily aroused. Now, in the analysis, it was becoming possible to visualise the dual reality in which the patient lived: that of the analytic relationship, which was beneficial to her, and the parallel reality of her secret fantasy life, on which she placed such high value.

The dissociated fantasy life has always been present in the patient. In her memories of childhood, the glory days were when her father— even if he was taciturn and had a cruel streak, especially towards animals—took her riding with him. On those occasions, she could dream of being his privileged companion, and was seemingly aroused by the mere fact of being an object of desire. In the dream, this is evidently the mutual aim of both protagonists, analyst and patient.

This type of erotic transference manifestly betrayed the existence in this patient of a profound sense of desolation and lack of personal meaning. She plainly used love, whether divulged or cultivated in fantasy, as a compensation for this underlying void.

A suitable way of escaping from this painful sense of non-existence seemed to her to be, precisely, the creation of a fantasied erotic reality, which she would then think of as real. The awareness arrived at through her therapy of the falsification she had applied to her life enabled her to achieve greater integration, thus conferring meaning on her life in reality.

The sexualised transference

Sexualisation is not only a defence mechanism, otherwise it would be impossible to explain why it can become a stable, anti-relational psychopathological structure that eventually holds sway over the patient's internal world.

An excellent example of this process is given by Meltzer (1966) in his description of anal masturbation. His model is that of a baby who tries to avoid the perception of anxiety as the mother walks away by idealising his own bottom; the arousal obtained from the anal mastur-bation obliterates the perception of loss and replaces it with a sexual short-circuit.

Meltzer (1973) also describes the process of mental sexualisation occurring in certain psychotic states, perversions, and cases of drug dependency. Here the patient succeeds in creating a masturbatory state of arousal that distances him from reality; the transformation is so pleasurable that he is unaware of the dangers of the process and, therefore, fails to ask for help.

Sexualisation corresponds to a withdrawal of the mind into the aroused body, and is characteristic of the perverse mental state. The psychopathological organisation offers seemingly irresistible perverse pleasures.

In the sexualised erotic transference, which I describe as *malignant*, the patient attempts to draw the analyst into the same mental state.

Some aspects of this situation are illustrated by the following clin-ical vignette from the first two years of the analysis of a young female patient who brought a particularly prolonged sexualised transference into the analytic relationship.

* * *

Before her analysis, the patient, Aurelia, had been living with a young man who used drugs, and had given birth to a little girl by him. While she herself resorted to drugs sporadically, he was a persistent user and eventually died of an overdose. At the beginning of the therapy, Aurelia appeared worried and depressed, but, after about a year of analysis, the atmosphere between us changed unexpectedly. Aurelia seemed to have forgotten all her suffering, including her partner's death, and felt constantly aroused—which she experienced as a return to "life". In the transference, on the other hand, I was seen as too "slow" and "conformist", and was often the target of provocative com-ments that ridiculed both myself and the analysis. At this point, she began to make manifest, unequivocal, and insistent sexual advances. Sometimes, on arriving for her session, Aurelia, instead of lying down on the couch, would even stretch out on the floor and make as if to undress. When, of course, I asked her not to do so, she would comment sarcastically on my timidity and hypocrisy. On other occasions she would extol the virtues of a drug and offer me a small dose. During this period, Aurelia did indeed appear to be drugged herself, the predominant drug being the sexualisation of her mind. In the counter-transference, I felt disturbed and worried. I was disturbed because I felt, so to speak, bombarded, exposed to constant projective identifica-tion, intended by the patient to change my mental state and to trans-port me into her own state of arousal, and worried because Aurelia was not only acting out in her sessions, but also indulging in increas-ingly violent and dangerous promiscuous sexual activity outside.

I was convinced that a sexualised, drug-addicted nucleus was trying to destroy the analysis, presenting it as a banal and hypocriti-cal relationship that was worthless in comparison with the sexual pleasure we could have achieved together. The struggle was waged not only between herself and myself, but also, and in particular, between two different parts of the patient, as the sexualised part sought to take possession of her healthy part.

Therefore, I did my best, in the analytic work, to support her healthy part in order to release it from the power of the sexualised part. After a long period of such work, this aggressive, violent sexu-ality, which often frightened her in her dreams and waking fantasies, gradually became less virulent.

This period of the analysis ended with a dream that marked the point when the patient succeeded in more consciously escaping from this sexualised madness:

> "In what felt like a science-fiction movie, I was looking for a house with my daughter. A couple of friends pointed one out to me, but when I approached it I saw that it was actually a grave, with a white-painted casket; the only way to live in it was to lie down inside having sex with a man. I decided not to go in because I realised that if I did I'd lose my daughter for ever."

* * *

The dream represents a form of sexualisation that is clearly symbol-ised as very dangerous: the sexualised object, which is capable of capturing the patient's self, displays an uncanny face. The patient becomes aware that this repetitive, greedy sexuality risks swallowing her up once and for all, dragging her off into an irreversible deadly mental state. The dream betrays an awareness that remained unconscious until it was worked through within the analytic relationship.

In other words, complex analytic work enabled the patient to distinguish clearly between what seemed to her good because it aroused her and gave her pleasure (something that was now proving to be destructive) and what was remote from pleasure but was actually constructive and relational (in this case, the bond with her daughter).

An erotic transference that includes a powerful sexual component in which "the logic of soup, with dumplings for arguments" is prevalent differs from an idealising loving transference. Here, the patient's declaration completely lacks the dreamlike, gentle aspect described above in connection with the idealising loving transference. Seduction, or the attempted projection of arousal on to the partner, is characterised by constant pressure and, instead of giving rise to any positive feelings in the analyst, induces in him an unpleasurable emotion. This is because the strength of the projection is likely to suggest to the analyst that what is involved is a delusional idea, if the idea is delusional partly on account of its capacity to monopolise, attract to itself, and dissolve any other idea, thus causing it to appear as false.

Under the pressure of the patient's projection and in the climate of unreality that forms, the analyst feels powerless in the face of the "dumplings for arguments", and must fight against the annoying sense that his belief in his analytic skill or in the existence of analysis is nothing but an illusion on which he has fed. The analyst is exposed by the patient to the delusional experience of hallucination, and the patient's illusory power is wielded precisely by the attempt to undermine the analyst's sense of his analytic identity.

The patient, after all, needs to transport the analyst, too, into the Garden of Eden; the state aimed for in relation to the object appears similar to a temporary alteration of consciousness, replete with mutual, false identifications.

This state differs from an actual psychosis in that a psychotic ultimately believes that his erotised world (usually centred on his own body) can sever any link of dependence between himself and the outside world; in our case, by contrast, the patient depends on, and searches for, suggestible and dependent objects. In seeking a convertible or suggestible object in the analyst, the omnipotence of the fantasy of fascination can readily lead the patient to believe that he has turned the analyst into an object that really is seducible. If the analyst actually does act out or is assumed to do so by the patient, even in relation to something as seemingly banal as a change of session time, this might intensify the patient's arousal and be interpreted by him as meaning that he has achieved his purpose.

The point, however, is that the analyst is seen as a potentially arousable interlocutor (who is, moreover, easily interchangeable with other partners in the patient's life) who can and must share the illusory world projected on to him by the patient.

The analyst's confusion about his identity is, in fact, a token of the patient's dilemma: he does not know whether he is a sexual adult or a small child aroused by his own omnipotence.

I contend that *sexualisation of the analytic relationship* does not involve a potential for emotional development, and should be considered very differently in analysis from an idealising loving transference. A sexualised transference of this kind should be treated as a psychopathological structure that seeks to colonise the analysand's mind. Interpretations should aim to help the patient escape from the power of the psychopathological structure by describing its nature and working in alliance with the healthy part of the patient.

My technique with Aurelia, intended primarily to release her from the confusion and seductive power wielded over her by the pathological object, can be seen as one of the possible therapeutic approaches.

In the malignant transference, the patient's attitude is, as a rule, characterised by a deep-seated failure to understand the nature and colonising power of this mental state: the sexualised exaltation presents itself to the patient as a pleasurable and desirable solution and is put forward as such to the analyst, too.

Notwithstanding patients' explicit belief in the goodness of this mental state, it is not difficult to apprehend in their dreams a representation of the uncanny, anxiety-inducing, and deadly character of this dependence, as encountered in the case of Aurelia.

The delusional transference

So far, I have described some configurations of the complex entity of the erotic transference. The most unfavourable outcome of this mental state is its transformation into a delusional transference.

The word "daydreams" can be used to denote secretly cultivated fantasies that coexist, or are maintained in parallel, with an individual's relational reality and everyday life. However, the point may sometimes come when the balance between the two realities is shifted in favour of the one constructed in the imagination. If that occurs, the dissociated reality takes over, obliterates the perception of psychic reality, and becomes a delusion.

The delusional state can be seen as a falsification undertaken in the imagination, of which the patient is unaware, and which imposes itself on consciousness, thus progressively distorting the sense of reality.

Delusion differs, by virtue of its concrete character, from other forms of imagination such as daydreams, the fantasies of infancy, or play, of which defensive aspects, curiosity, or exploration of the world are important components. In other words, there is a qualitative difference between the positive forms of imagination needed to keep the future open or to construct new shared realities, on the one hand (as in the ideal loving transference), and delusional falsifications, on the other (as in sexualised or delusional transferences). The delusional state is the outcome of a prolonged psychic withdrawal in which the organs of perception are used to generate artificial states of well-being. That is what happens in the delusional loving transference.

* * *

I had an experience of this kind with my patient Maria. When her therapy began, she was not delusional, had not had psychotic episodes, and did not exhibit any obvious symptoms of such a state. I had learnt from her that she had in the past fallen unhappily in love with older men—and once even with a priest—but I had, unfortunately, not foreseen that this situation would be repeated with the force of a delusion.

In my analytic experience until then, a dream or an allusion had sufficed to warn me in time of the onset of an incipient erotic transference, thus allowing me to intervene so as to steer the analysis in the right direction. However, no such communication had been forthcoming in Maria's therapy; instead, we often had to confront a painful attachment that made analytic separations difficult and traumatic. I saw Maria as a deprived and depressed person, but not as someone with psychotic propensities, as subsequently proved to be the case.

A few months into the analysis, the patient brought a dream that I did not understand until the erotic transference emerged a few years later.

> In the dream the patient was with a group of people and then decided to take the elevator by herself to a higher level, but on arrival found that she could no longer operate the controls and remained incarcerated in the elevator.

* * *

At the time, nothing was further from my mind than the thought—which only occurred to me much later—that the dream might represent an ascent into psychosis (the elevator obviously described a manic state) from which the patient was afraid she would never be able to emerge. For a long time I had thought that Maria was suffering from a form of melancholic depression; this seemed obvious to me from the type of aggressive, painful attachment displayed in the transference. Her history featured a childhood and adolescence afflicted by an aggressive and violent mother, the father having died early on. Although I thought that this infantile experience had burdened the patient's development, every attempt to put her in touch with the suffering of her infancy had failed.

In the course of time, Maria developed a delusional relationship with me, as became obvious in her project to marry me. This intention was not a dream—it lacked the relevant emotional and symbolic aspect—but an objective that she pursued concretely and in full awareness. Her "dreams", on the other hand, went unmentioned by the patient; in fact, she maintained a stubborn silence about these entities, which were actually daydreams of an intensely illusory nature, for Maria had decided not to disclose these "dreams" to me lest they were destroyed by my unwillingness to share them.

At any rate, they were not like the dreams of a neurotic patient trying to communicate the nature of her emotions to herself and the analyst. Instead, they were newly created realities that were doggedly cherished by the patient and had to be protected at all costs.

Maria's "dreams" were not really dreams at all. Rather than metaphorical representations, they were realities from which Maria derived a particular narcissistic pleasure. Neither were they bearers of an unconscious meaning to be uncovered; their meaning was manifest, clear, and concrete, and, for that reason, they were exciting and seductive.

One of the complex and paradoxical aspects of the analytic therapy of psychosis is that for long periods the "psychotic part" is absent, invisible, or impossible to apprehend, and, when it does emerge, it does so unexpectedly when the psychotic transformation has already occurred. It seems to me that, in her analysis, Maria had for a long time kept secret a world dissociated from reality and that the dissociated reality had ultimately taken over and become a delusion.

When the decision to marry me emerged into the light, I at first treated it as a symptom to be analysed, but, as a result, Maria's relationship with me became increasingly stormy. In her exasperation, the patient said she wanted to break off the analysis and to consult a woman analyst with a view to undertaking a new therapy.

> After one such consultation, she brought me a dream in which she was a guest in my female colleague's garden in a marvellous, timeless atmosphere; but then everything was interrupted by an attendant, who took it upon himself to close the gate and put an end to the rendezvous.

This dream clearly showed that the patient hated me for attempting to put an end to her delusion—which she was, however, skilfully hiding—while already rebuilding it in the lateral transference with my colleague. It also emerged from the dream that the enchanted garden corresponded to an experience from her infancy that she had never mentioned to me. Quite often, her maternal grandmother would take Maria with her to a villa in the country where they would spend months on end together, the two of them withdrawn from the world, and the patient had no desire to go back to school to see her friends again. I believe that this seduction by the grandmother, who transported her into an ideal, timeless atmosphere (in effect, a psychosis à deux), had laid the foundations for her search for a special, delusional condition with me.

Maria's material, as reported above, is also clinically important in that the character of her "dreams" offered an insight into how her psychotic part, when no longer contained, had overcome the rest of her personality.

Maria did not go into analysis with my female colleague, who did not have a place for her, but chose another male analyst. I later heard that she had had three manifestly psychotic episodes—all with delusional sexual content—for which she had been hospitalised.

The benign and malignant transference

As a general rule, it is, in my view, possible to draw a useful clinical distinction between the *benign* loving transference and the *malignant* sexual transference.

The benign loving transference is represented by the cases of Madeleine, reported above, who developed an idealised love relationship with me after a period of emotional distance. In the analytic process in this case, the unforeseen blaze of emotion was usually followed by periods of silence. The work of therapy involved keeping this relationship alive so as to allow it to develop.

A similar situation is described by Gould (1994): after initial disorientation and countertransference difficulties with a male patient's stormy loving transference, the analyst realised its potential for development and responded with empathy. This gave rise to an important change: the initial love-based "siege" was transformed into a deep emotional bond helpful to the progress of the analysis.

Owing to its potential for development, it would be inappropriately reductive to analyse it in terms of a resistance to the relationship of analytic dependence. Neither does it seem correct to interpret the loving transference as a reactivation of the past in the present, as this might well be construed by the patient as a defence by the analyst against the formation of a bond that concerns him personally. In his essay, Freud (1915a) leaves the matter unresolved, stressing the transformative power of transference love—a force "impelling [the patient] to . . . make changes"—and not merely its defensive or regressive character.

The benign loving transference does not excessively disturb the analyst, who is called upon to share an ideal, infantile type of experience. He must be capable of calibrating his response in such a way as to avoid interfering with the development of the patient's experience and, as far as possible, to support that experience. This type of transference is indicative of the patient's initial capacity to *dream* an affective relationship and demonstrates his entry into an emotional and relational world.

The sexualised transference, on the other hand, may give rise to a countertransference response that is not at all easily controllable. Whereas, in the loving transference, the patient wants to experience an emotional state with the analyst, in the sexual transference he aspires to change the analyst's mind. Such stubborn and violent manipulation often results in a countertransference response of alarm or rejection.

If sexuality proper is distinguished from its pathological version (that is, sexualisation), even certain early infantile sexual manifestations—for example, in children who will later develop a perversion (De Masi, 2003[1999])—must be seen as anomalous, abnormal components of sexuality.

For if a child does not obtain emotional responses favourable to mental growth from his primary objects, he will try to sustain himself by forms of arousal that amount to actual sexual withdrawal. This situation recurs in the sexual transference: the analysand distances himself from the relational experience by resorting to forms of arousal or masturbatory activity. While this process may be encouraged by deficiencies in the analyst's analytic function, it may also be observed in their absence.

This involves a vicious circle similar to that seen in the perversions, in which, mixed with the sense of desperation, a sexualised object is idealised and set up against the absent love relationship. The sexualised transference is located inside this vicious circle, and one of the analyst's tasks is to remove it from the circle. The timing of interpretation is all-important: it must be appropriate and continuous, especially in the case of a delusional transference, so as to prevent the psychotic nucleus from colonising the rest of the personality (Rosenfeld, 2001).

A complementarity between the mental states described here—idealisation, erotisation, and malignant sexualisation—can now be glimpsed, if only in their discontinuity. The more the relationship of mutual receptivity in analysis fails, the weaker the element of idealising protection becomes, while, at the same time, the sexualised or perverse aspect is potentiated, thus causing the patient to lapse from the initial erotised relationship into a form of sexualised madness.

The sexualised transference is feared by patients themselves, owing to its tantalising character. Analysis with a man might ultimately prove impossible with some female patients, who may, if at all, turn to a woman analyst instead.

The arousal generated by this "other" (dissociated) reality also explains why the sexual transference might be imperceptibly transformed into an actual delusion, as in the case of Maria, described above.

Furthermore, any sexual acting out by the analyst—aside from ethical considerations—is, of course, likely to prove catastrophic for the patient. In the case of an idealising loving transference, the analyst, with his desire, occupies his analysand's *potential space for development*, thus rendering it unavailable to the analysand, whose onward path will ultimately be blocked thereby. In an overtly sexualised transference situation, the analyst eventually finds himself in the same regressive position as his patient, whose pathological part thereby triumphs over the now irremediably defeated healthy part.

The patient's basic structure (depressive, hysterical, borderline, or psychotic) probably correlates with the quality of the erotic transference. The more severe and deep-rooted the pathological structure, the fewer the possibilities of emotional development in the transference and the more difficult the transformation of that structure will be.

As I have attempted to show in my clinical examples, every form of human sexuality and love may be encountered in this type of transference, ranging from tender, intimate, and gentle love resembling a dreamlike state, via overwhelming passion, to a level of arousal that makes sexuality as compulsive as an addictive drug.

Within this complex, multi-faceted spectrum, the analyst must find his bearings and constantly switch between elements of development and regression, in order to lead the patient sustainably into the realm of emotional relating and mental growth.

CHAPTER TEN

Is it possible to cure paedophilia?[*]

"As a boy-lover, I don't seek out boys for my personal pleasure.
I simply encourage those that come to me and want to play
sexy games with me; I've always seen it like this. I've never
been violent towards a boy"

(Declaration of a seventy-four-year-old paedophile)

P aedophilia inherently conserves the feature of being ego-
syntonic; in other words, the perversion is not seen by the
subject as being something conflictual or blameful. Paedophile
patients do not generally arrive spontaneously in analysis, and, when
they do, it is not easy for the therapist to have any clear idea about
how to proceed with the treatment. This chapter attempts to describe
the nature of this morbid condition, and illustrates an analytic therapy
carried out successfully.

---

* First published in *The International Journal of Psychoanalysis, 88*: 147–165 with the title
"The paedophile and his inner world: theoretical and clinical considerations on the
analysis of a patient. Translated by Giovanna Iannaco.

"The only respectable thing about my life is my birth. The rest is unpublishable." This is what Norman Douglas, the twentieth-century English writer who settled in Capri, declared to his biographer. Douglas was referring to his attraction for young boys and his love for one of them, with whom he had cohabited for a long time. Another declaration of his had been: "Surround yourself with children and adolescents, only this keeps the mind young". For the paedophile (and Douglas was one) the child is, indeed, not only a sexualised being, but also an object which brings energy and vitality (Lowenfels, 1962).

Paedophilia: classical times and the contemporary era

It is well known that in some historical eras some cultures admitted paedophilia. This could even take a ritualised and institutionalised form. In classical Greece, sexual relations between adult and adolescent males were frequent within contexts of spiritual and pedagogical development. While homosexual love for the adolescent was allowed, promiscuous homosexuality of a pornographic or mercenary nature was punished (Cantarella, 1992). Similarly, sexual relations with prepubescent children were severely punished: the boy involved in a sexual relationship could not be younger than twelve years old. The phenomenon of "socially accepted" paedophilia disappeared with the world of ancient Greece. It is now completely alien to us, because of the profound transformation of the adult–child relationship over time and also because of shifts in the conception of sexuality and of generational differences.

Regarding paedophilia as a modern problem, it is important to underline that what seems to be a new phenomenon, characteristic of our age, is actually the social organisation of paedophilia (and of perversion in general) rather than the underlying mental structure. What is new about paedophilia is its conspicuousness. On the Internet, there are sites offering products tailored to the tastes and preferences of the customer. Paedophile organisations, just like their counterparts dealing with other forms of perversion, aspire to emerge from the clandestine so as to communicate freely and obtain validation and consent. This kind of self-promotion has the aim of dissolving the solitary nature of paedophilia and, by rendering legitimate the sexual choice of the adepts, of erasing the transgressive motive and subsequent liability.

Currently, paedophilia is a widespread phenomenon with entrenched financial and tourist interests. The encounter between the industrialised western world and the developing countries allows the childhood of the poor and vulnerable to be violated on a systematic and global scale. Television reports show us little girls sold by their parents in remote rural areas, or young boys compliantly prostituting themselves. Precociously burned out by their struggle for survival in the cities, they offer their bodies to groups of westerners whose pockets are full of money.

Another characteristic of contemporary paedophilia is the volume of erotic and pornographic material in circulation, ranging from publishing to video production. The conspicuousness of paedophile behaviour and the increased attention given to it by the media and public opinion (consider events in the Roman Catholic Church in the USA and, more recently, in Brazil) suggest a likely future demand for psychoanalytic treatment also for this kind of disturbance. This work aims to be a contribution to possible clinical experiences in the field.

Paedophilia and psychoanalysis

Freud seems to have considered paedophilia more as an occasional act than as a perversion as such. In his *Three Essays on the Theory of Sexuality* (1905d), he states that children are substitute objects for those who are not able to have a sexual relationship with other partners: only exceptionally are they the exclusive object (p. 146). His early clinical cases abound with episodes of child seduction by servants, nannies, or relatives. It is this that might have induced him to reason that the origin of neurosis is seated in early sexual trauma.

One of the reasons for the paucity of analytical literature on this subject is that paedophiles very rarely ask spontaneously for therapy. Even the treatments prescribed following conviction are accepted only as alternatives preferable to a sentence. Now, a therapy which is not freely chosen and which does not allow for deep and systematic interrelating, often keeps the paedophile area split and encapsulated. Thus, even in the presence of some improvement in some aspects of the personality, such therapies do not guarantee that paedophile behaviour will not recur.

Definitions

First of all, there is the problem of how to consider paedophilia. Can the paedophile act be unique, an exceptional event that has nothing to do with the whole personality of the person who commits it? Or does it derive from the structure of the personality and tend to repeat itself? Is the paedophile capable also of having a sexual relationship with an adult, and of leading an apparently normal married life, or is he entirely dedicated to an erotic relationship with a child?

Does the act of sexual abuse by the paedophile on the child always imply violence, tending, at the extreme, to criminal aggression? Or is it necessary to make some distinctions between criminal sexual aggression on minors (as can be made with criminal sexual aggression on women) and true paedophilia, which, in itself, is far from any violence? Sexual abuse of the under-aged is not always synonymous with paedophilia, but can stem from other psychopathological conditions (such as schizophrenia and mental deterioration). In these cases, we talk of secondary paedophilia.

In a study at an Italian psychiatric hospital (Jaria, 1969), almost half of the 156 patients who had abused minors were mentally disabled. The next largest group were schizophrenics, then alcoholics, and, finally, people with mental disorders due to old age. It is clear that such statistics record numbers of people sentenced and who are not, therefore, representative of the true paedophile. The latter usually manage to avoid criminal prosecution, being highly skilled in avoiding the legal consequences of their acts.

It is also important to distinguish true paedophilia from the sexual violations that happen within a family. Despite the fact that there are profound analogies between these two conditions (they both ignore the incest taboo and the difference between generations), the parent who abuses his daughter or son is sometimes in a regressive position due to a real psychopathological condition. Glasser (1988) is right to remark that incest implies complex intrafamiliar dynamics that are completely alien to paedophilia.

Paedophilia can be divided into two forms: the *structured* and the *occasional*. When the sexual objects are exclusively children or adolescents, we talk of structured paedophilia, which can be either hetero- or homosexual. If the paedophile leads an apparently normal life and has sexual relationships also with adults, we talk of occasional paedophilia. In this case, there is also a certain degree of awareness and of guilt about the paedophile act. However, even in the occasional forms observed in psychotherapy, in which the sexual act seems to have been committed under conditions of stress, the existence of a paedophile imaginary world can be discerned under a façade of an apparently normal sexuality (Glasser, 1988). Socarides (1959) believes that occasional paedophilia is more prevalent in middle age or at the onset of old age, when important psychological changes alter the defences against sexual impulses.

Paedophilia can occur on its own or combined with other perversions, the most dangerous being sadism. Taking into account this last aspect, I tend to distinguish between two forms of paedophilia: the *romantic* and the *cynical*.

"Romantic" paedophilia is nurtured by the eroticised and idealised figure of a little boy or girl. Norman Douglas, James Barrie (author of *Peter Pan*, 1995), and Lewis Carroll (*Alice's Adventures in Wonderland*, 1971) could be examples of this kind of paedophilia. The world of the "romantic" paedophile is, in fact, centred on the life of young people, both for its affective and for its imagined erotic aspects: the desired object is more often an adolescent than a child. This does not mean that this form of paedophilia is limited to the sublimation of sexuality: it always culminates in a concrete sexual approach.

One famous literary example of "romantic" paedophilia is found in Nabokov's *Lolita* (1959), in which a lonely and melancholic university lecturer falls passionately in love with an adolescent girl. In describing the encounter between the erotic dependence of the adult and the cynicism of the adolescent, Nabokov establishes an ambiguity around the role of the victim. The girl, who has grown up too quickly in a cynical, middle-class environment, appears much more resilient than the academic, who is completely defenceless and enslaved to his own passion. In this form of paedophiliac love, the adult, too, can end up as the dominated victim.

In "cynical" paedophilia, the underlying fantasy is sadistic: a state of mental excitement is only reached through imagining maltreatment or violence on the child. The pleasure does not derive from sexual desire, but, rather, from being able to do anything one wishes to a submissive object. The child is more liable than others to become the object of criminal sadistic fantasies. Often this aim is achieved through the use of pictures or videos from the illegal paedophile pornographic trade.

It is legitimate to wonder whether sadism is an avoidable factor or whether it is an intrinsic part of the perverse structure of paedophilia. From a psychodynamic perspective, it is possible to intuit why sexuality addressed to children can be a fertile ground for sadism: the child is desirable because submissive and psychologically defenceless. In fact, the asymmetrical relationship (adult–child, dominant–dominated) that characterises the paedophile perversion can experience a dramatic escalation towards sadistic arousal. Even so, paedophilia, while characterised by an asymmetrical relationship, an aspect also seen in sadomasochism, does not necessarily lead to the pleasure of sadistic violence. This is why it is necessary to make a distinction between the forms of criminal sexuality on children and adolescents and paedophilia as such, which, in itself, is far from violence. Even though the paedophile sexual act is always an abuse, "romantic" paedophiles often show altruistic features or educational and creative skills in their relationship with the children. This contrasts with "sadistic" paedophiles who have no relationship with the children and are not in the least fascinated by the world of childhood.

Characteristics of the paedophile world

In paedophilia, the relationship is "asymmetric". Paedophile love can be seen as a defence against relating with an object perceived as independent.

Idealisation of the body of a child or adolescent is matched by an aversion to the physical aspect and to the psychic and emotional world of the adult. As soon as the child shows any sign of secondary sexual features, the rapid and unexpected rise of the adult physical form destroys the idealisation of childish beauty.

The paedophile wants to be a boy and to mix with other boys in a world of playfulness and imagination. Just like Peter Pan, he wants to stop time and to realise the myth of eternal youth. This explains why the paedophile tends to choose professions that allow a constant immersion in the world of childhood or adolescence. For the paedophile imagination, parents do not exist: the child is a *puer beatus*, self-generated and totally self-sufficient.

Paedophiles often had an isolated childhood. As children, they felt excluded by their peers and envied their vitality. As adults, they desire to possess those very children they admired and envied. The loving and sexual relationship with the child or adolescent also expresses a fantasy of recovering a lost or never possessed vitality. Who does not remember the writer Aschenbach, his creativity blocked and tormented by the idea of getting old, falling in love with the adolescent Tadzio in Thomas Mann's *Death in Venice* (1995)? While claiming to be the only people capable of understanding children or adolescents, "romantic" paedophiles distort the world of children because they sexualise it: the child's warmth and intimacy are often misunderstood as an invitation to sex.

In the case of paedophilia, the sexualisation of psychic reality could be due to early trauma or sexual abuses. However, it is often the case that the adult paedophile has not been the young victim of sexual violence; he might, on the contrary, have been privileged or have been the object of psychological seductions on the part of one or both parents. It is not unusual for paedophiles to have been intelligent, sensitive, and privileged children who had an enchanted childhood, which they emerged from traumatically following a loss of trust in their parents. Subsequently, they sought refuge in a sexualised world, seen as a continuous source of arousal and support. The experience of an infantile sexualised withdrawal determines the unconscious belief of the paedophile that all children are "naturally" desirous of sexual experiences. The patient described by Arundale (1999) claimed that his most fervent wish was to make children happy and he daydreamed of a happy country in which it was permissible to have sexual relationships with them.

I now want to say something about the origin of perversion in general and of paedophilia in particular. Perverse behaviours find their roots in infancy. They express a dependency on a state of mental excitement that must absolutely not be confused with the exertion of relational sexuality. Sexuality, which is present in the paedophile perversion, is sustained by fantasies that are self-generated in a state of psychic withdrawal. This state alters the perception of psychic and emotive reality and has an addictive quality. Thus, the paedophile sees in the child and in the adolescent someone who desires sexuality and who constantly proposes themselves as a sexual object. Devious sexual behaviour often stems from early infancy in abandoned, deprived, or isolated children. These children take refuge in a fantasised, sexualised world. It is this state of mind that, later on, combined with the disillusion caused by the adult world and with a reluctance to grow up, will sustain that person's evolution towards paedophilia.

An analytic therapy

I now present a paedophile homosexual patient, whose paedophile fantasies are tightly interwoven with sadistic and masochistic ones. Analytic therapy, conducted at a rate of four weekly sessions, began fourteen years ago and is now coming to an end. In this chapter, I focus mainly on the nature of the pathological structure underlying this patient's paedophilia and describe the transformation that occurred in analysis. The perspective I propose underlines the specific nature of the analytic work with this kind of patient and seeks to determine what needs to be analysed in the first place. By this, I am not intending to make an artificial distinction between a true analytic cure (which is based on the transference and countertransference dynamic, the interpretation of fantasies, and of pathological identifications, and so on) and the cure of the "paedophile nucleus". As previously described, I consider the world of paedophilia to be determined by a sexualised nucleus, split from the rest of the personality, which is constantly trying to seduce the healthy part of the patient.

The main analytic task is to help the patient to neutralise the power of this pathological structure. The analyst will be constantly drawn into the patient's sexualised world, which is at the basis of paedophilia. Within the dreams and fantasies belonging to this world, he will progressively come to represent, in the transference, the parental figures of the past, the patient's internal objects or a new figure who can facilitate the development of the healthier part of the patient.

*   *   *

Michele is a thirty-year-old man whose objects of sexual attraction are children or prepubescent boys. He dedicates his professional time to them, as a teacher, and as much as possible of his free time. He is truly attracted by children and adolescents and finds a nourishing pleasure in their company. Despite the presence of perverse fantasies which have, as an object, adolescents with whom he identifies, the idealisation of the world of childhood and adolescence makes Michele more of a "romantic" than a "cynical" paedophile. However, I believe that, without analytic help, even the 'romantic" part of Michele would sooner or later have given way to the "cynical" component.

His sadomasochistic fantasies go back to his early infancy. He remembers how, as a little child he could reach states of mental orgasm through fantasies based on stories of submission, injuries, and pain. His homosexuality established itself during adolescence. At that time, he started to feel sexually attracted by his peers. He has never had a real relationship, and, on the occasions of a few attempts, he has found himself to be impotent. The attraction towards paedophilia was perhaps meant to be a solution to this failure: when he was about twenty-five years old he attempted to sexually seduce his pre-adolescent brother and fell in love with the ten-year-old son of a neighbour. In childhood, a privileged relationship with his mother placed him in a special position in relation to his siblings (an elder sister, two sisters and two brothers younger than him). In adolescence, this relationship deteriorated as the mother, also attracted by the adolescent world, developed an idealised bond with a boy of Michele's age. Michele also found this boy very handsome and desirable. From then on, the patient, full of rage, distanced himself from his mother. At the time, his relationship with his father was already very troubled. After early childhood, apparently free from conflict, his father had tried to educate him in an authoritarian way, pushing him towards a position of rebellious submission, mixed with feelings of fear and persecution. Despite the fact that Michele is now an adult able to take an intellectual and professional role in the social sphere, he has no significant contact with adults. He constantly seeks to meet children and adolescents (strictly males only) and dedicates himself to setting up playgroups in which he has the role of facilitator. These same children and boys are the object of his sexualised fantasies.

The perception of his isolation and the fear of becoming completely dominated by his paedophile and sexual fantasies pushed him to ask for analytic help. I recall one of his first dreams in analysis:

"A child is kidnapped and taken to the brothels of South-East Asia. On his return, he appears completely transformed: he looks brain damaged, like an idiot; he seems to have Down's syndrome."

The content of this dream highlights the patient's anxiety of not being able to control his sexualised arousal (the brothel), perceived as an irreversibly destructive occurrence for the mind. For a long period in analysis, the sessions are dominated by sexual, sadomasochistic, and paedophilic fantasies, described in minute detail. A typical fantasy, with many variations, is the one in which a homosexual relationship between an adult and a young boy is transformed into a sadomasochistic relationship in which the patient, identified with both partners, draws pleasure from the active acquiescence of the boy and from the sadistic initiatives of the adult. This kind of fantasy, not in the least masked, appears also in dreams, which are not dissimilar from the constructions made by the patient in the wakeful state. For long periods, the consulting room is literally invaded by dreams set in dark caves, peopled by monstrous figures; primitive animals are ridden in crescendos of arousal, while children are frantically stripped of their clothes, penetrated, or made objects of sadistic violence.

It is during this first period that Michele develops with me a polemical and aggressive transference. In particular, I become the object of malignant projections and of fierce criticism for being unable to think and for my arrogant, adult narcissism.

*   *   *

If I were to frame the analytical relationship of the first years of this analysis from the perspective of the perverse transference, I should say that Michele is using a consolidated technique that consists in projecting into his interlocutor irritation and rage to the point of provoking in the latter a counter-aggressive reaction. As soon as he feels that the desired effect has been achieved, he becomes cold and rational and, from his achieved superiority, he can stigmatise the behaviour of the other. In this aggressive way of relating, he always finds someone to whom to attribute responsibility and blame: in the past, it was his parents, and now it is the analyst in the transference. He also comes into conflict with other people in his everyday life. If they happen to have an authoritative role, they become for him persecutors whom he hates and whom he provokes with an ostentatious display of innocence.

During the sessions, he shows a distinctive ability to isolate single sentences of mine from the context. Once separated and distorted, the sentence will appear to him particularly obscure, stupid, and offensive. Having found a blatant element of offence on my part, he can voice his polemic. As an analytical victim, he has the right to attack and beat me pitilessly. As is easy to imagine, this countertransference knot is not always easy to undo. Michele seems to have a particular ability to create between him and the other a climate of irritated mistrust. Perception of the interlocutor's silent or defensive response is the starting point for a new attack. I must say that, of all my patients, he is the one who has most strongly tested my counter-transference stamina. To give a brief example of the perverse way in which Michele tends to transform the other into a bad object while putting himself in the position of the innocent victim, I describe the way he responded on one occasion when I announced to him that I had to cancel one session. Not in the least disappointed, Michele asks me the reasons for this cancellation. I let him know the reasons (joinery works next door to my consulting room, which will render the session impossible because of the transport of materials as well as noise), but he says that he is not satisfied and insists several times on my giving more information about the works. When I reply that in my opinion he has received enough information, he rebels, attacking me and accusing me of denying him knowledge and of inhibiting his curiosity.

A delicate problem in Michele's analysis is represented by the choice of how to respond to him: the understanding of his mental state must include a firm position that challenges his arrogant assertion of himself over others (and, in the transference, over myself) and, at the same time, analyses the continuous attack upon the potential positive dependence on a human object. Although they originate in traumatic past experiences, the resentment and the spite in the trans-ference also represent an attack on parental figures as such. In other words, resentment and spite have the role of sustaining the idea, cen-tral to paedophilia and to perversion in general, that parents do not exist, or, if they do, are denigrated and degraded objects (Chasseguet-Smirgel, 1985). The attacks on parents (and on the analyst in the trans-ference) serve the purpose of justifying and idealising the paedo-phile world, seen as superior to any other. Despite his conscious rage at the betrayal and the unreliability of his mother, the patient shares the same fantasy world. Just like her, he is fascinated by the world of male adolescents. He is sexually attracted by it and, like her, he would like to seduce handsome boys. However, Michele is not at all willing to consider the evident fact of his identification with his mother: any interpretation in this sense provokes irritation and anger.

Sexualisation

The dreams and the accounts of the patient are constantly coloured by sexualisation. In one dream in the patient's third year of analysis, *he is with a little boy. They are clasped together and rolling in the snow.* The patient experiences sexual pleasure: the docility of the child arouses him, his pleasure deriving from a sense of total union and adaptability on the part of the object. The coldness (the snow) and the malleability refer undoubtedly to the absence of emotions in the physical interpenetration. Thus, the dream hints at the possibility of penetrating and annihilating the object by crushing him. This arouses the patient. The psychological "malleability" of his young partner confirms the patient's superiority in his own mind and his triumph over a submissive and controllable object.

In one of the following sessions, Michele talks about Nino, a young boy with whom he has been playing a board game. Nino wants to show his skill at the game. In the eyes of the patient, however, Nino is trying to put himself forward as a homosexual object of pleasure. A casual and fleeting touching of the hands becomes for the patient an implicit homosexual advance; he must reciprocate, for the young boy cannot be exposed to disappointment. For him, Nino is a source of pleasure and happiness. Paedophile homosexuality appears to him a revelation: it is the true dimension of life.

This sequence illustrates the extent to which the paedophile dimension has assumed the nature of an ecstatic revelation for Michele.

The patient talks about the adolescent group as though a self-contained entity, a monad full of balance and wisdom in which, for the main part, no outsider is needed for the exercise of sexuality. These wise and exceedingly good boys masturbate and have sex with each other. In the sexualised mental state of the patient, the boy becomes an object providing a continuous source of pleasure. He is equated to the penis, which is always at his disposal and readily aroused when stimulated. The erect penis of the boy can be sucked at will: all the homosexuals are fighting for it. The arousal of this sexual–oral infantile world of greediness promises the existence of an enchanted land of absolute and endless gratification. To keep the excitement alive and to fuel the pleasure, any inclination to love and care for the object must be annihilated and sacrificed in the name of triumph and possession. Arousal springs from the certainty of possessing the object of pleasure in an exclusive way, from the sense of domination in using it, including a certain dose of sadism in touching, pinching, and tormenting it, and in perceiving it as submissive to his commands.

In order to be able to draw pleasure from his fantasy, Michele must go far away from the world and from the presence of his parents and analyst. Their existence will lower the level of mental enthralment and the vividness of the perverse fantasy. The delusional nature of the paedophile withdrawal ("the other reality") becomes evident in some dreams that are authentic psychopathological constructions.

In one dream, for instance, his brother Antonio appears, whom the patient attempts to seduce erotically.

> "Antonio defends himself, pushing him away. Michele then 'materialises' a flying carpet and invites his brother to sit on it. The brother does so, becoming immobile and passive: now the patient can suck his erect penis."

The transformation performed by the patient with the "flying carpet" places the object in the "other" sexualised world and thrusts the patient into a dimension beyond reality.

In this dream, the *delusional* aspect specific to paedophilia is represented precisely by the transformation of the brother's figure. Initially pictured as an alive and independent person, the brother becomes a passive and sexualised object. This change happens through the use of the omnipotent instrument of fantasy (the flying carpet which, defying the reality principle, allows one to fly). In my opinion, this dream also shows the effects of sexualisation, which deadens the vitality and the autonomy of the object and of the patient himself.

Transformations in analysis

First phase

This period is characterised by the patient's relentless propaganda, aiming to impose on me the superiority of his perverse world. It also includes the most difficult countertransference moments. The patient often attacks me, not least because he sees in me a possible antagonist who could deprive him of a fantastic and excited world that brings him pleasure and the triumph of possession. In order to avoid the risk of being pulled in turn into the sadomasochistic circle, I try, in these instances, to keep in mind that Michele has been a suffering and ill child.

As I said earlier, the first part of the analysis is constantly dominated by the exciting power of paedophilic, sadomasochistic fantasies, appearing both in daydreams and in dreams. As soon as he starts analysis, Michele gives up masturbating, a habit that, in the past, had taken an exasperated compulsive form and had been present since his early childhood. During the entire first phase of the analysis, however, he uses the night-time dream to enter into the same masturbatory dimension that he denies himself in the waking state. During this period, the dream is not a "dreaming", but an "acting". Typically, his "dreams" reproduce a perverse paedophile scene culminating in a nocturnal emission. It is obvious that dreams of this kind do not refer symbolically to anything else: they are indeed actions (Segal, 1991).

However, even this sort of dream is important. Throwing light on his internal world, they allow me to describe to the patient his mental processes, in particular his conflicts and the attempts by his perverse component to seduce and overcome the healthy part. In this sense, even though the patient usually offers very few associations to his dreams, his dream production allows a constant visualisation of his mental functioning. Later on in the analysis, they will become an important vehicle of communication, highlighting the function that the analyst has in his internal world. Sometimes, they also clarify the nature of his changes of perspective and of his evolving processes.

In a session during the fifth year of analysis, Michele describes a holiday at his parents' home, where he felt marginalised and inferior in relation to his siblings, who were with their partners. Late in the evening, he takes refuge in the toilet, and, with a photo portraying adolescents, he constructs an arousing fantasy in which a satyr seduces a young boy. The world is transformed into this exclusively sexualised reality: he is possessed and conquered by this world.

In the following days, this exciting concoction stays with him, inflaming his mind and trapping him. In a session, the patient regrets having set off, once again, this perverse paedophile experience.

This last clinical vignette characterises one phase of the analysis in which the patient's wish to evade the power of the sexualised paedophile nucleus becomes evident. In this period, he starts to conceive the existence of a boy who does not masturbate, does not indulge in orgiastic activities, and maintains his mind open to contact with the world. In other words, a perceptive self starts to emerge that observes and enters into conflict with the sexualised part.

When the patient resists the fascination of the perverse paedophile part, the evidence of his masturbatory madness thrusts him into a state of despair. At the same time, the atmosphere in the analytic relationship changes. Attacks and polemics decrease: the patient seems to be less colonised by the world of perversion and less compelled, in the transference, to make polemical attacks on the parental figures.

Second phase

In the second phase of analysis (from the sixth year), a new configuration of the paedophile fantasy emerges: the construction of the boy-idol that I have already described in Chapter Six. I remember that Michele had brought a dream in which he had been unexpectedly abandoned by Rosario, a very vital adolescent with whom he had been playfully intimate.

This dream points to a fusion with an ideal object that is not a symbolic maternal substitute, but a fantasy object *in place of* the mother; the union is not eroticised, but represents a need for supporting the self and preventing him from falling into total despair. In the dream, the illusion of being self-sufficient and happy in worshipping the boy-idol is dashed and he feels accused by the idealised object of being the cause of his own misery. The idol, so the dream has it, requires total submission and devotion; if you lose it, you fall into despair and you are to blame.

Third phase

In this period, too, Michele is still spending most of his free time in the group of male adolescents, sharing their dreamy life and trying to be one of them. I realise that his search for relationships exclusively with boys is, at the same time, a way of reinforcing his male identity. In adolescence, Michele had excluded himself from his group of male peers and had stayed in contact only with female figures (his mother and some school girlfriends). He had, in his own words, "feminised" himself. Frequenting this group of boys, with its conflicts, uncertainties, and naïve beliefs, is also helping to decrease his idealisation of the adolescent world.

In this period, the analytical relationship is stronger: the patient increasingly turns to me as someone who can help him to know himself and understand the world. The sexualised fantasy appears sometimes, according to the vicissitudes of the transference and to moments of conflict. For instance, during a brief, unforeseen absence of mine, he dreams:

> he is searching paedophile sites on the Internet, but the analyst appears and protects him, while he perceives a tiny flame throwing light in the room.

The presence of the analyst in the paedophile world witnesses an increased permeability of the masturbatory withdrawal and allows for a certain degree of insight. The relapse into the paedophile fantasy also occurs in analogous situations of frustration. The new element, which is starting to make its appearance in the sessions, is the fact that the perverse fantasy can be gradually understood and deprived of its invasive power within the analytic hour.

The definite exit from the paedophile world coincides with his falling in love with a real, alive object: an eighteen-year-old boy. For the first time in his life, Michele experiences a loving relationship, free from sexualised fantasies, with a real and separate object. However, this first experience of being in love, kept secret, exposes him to a destabilising emotional turmoil. The loss of the boy, who at some point leaves him, causes a long period of psychic and physical pain, depression, and panic. The experience of pain and disillusion, shared in the analytic relationship, pushes Michele towards a more determined emancipation from the adolescent word. In fact, from that moment onwards he starts to value his relationships with adults, seen as more reliable and less disappointing than adolescents. In his friendships with his contemporaries, some female figures gradually appear.

Even though not completely eliminated, the power of the paedophile nucleus has greatly decreased. When the paedophile fantasy recurs, Michele is now able to link it to the object and to the emotional constellation that generated it. He can now understand its defensive or aggressive significance. The paedophile world is now felt as a residual element of the past. It cannot be removed from memory and could well become active again, but it appears well balanced and contained by the more insightful parts that the patient has developed. In the patient's words, it could only be reactivated in the presence of "bad masters"; that is, if he erased from the mind his links with emotional reality. In this case, he would become trapped once again in the claustrophiliac world of paedophilia.

However, Michele does not believe any longer in the poet of the Middle Ages who proclaims that being in the "castle with Ganymede" is preferable to normal sexuality.

Specific traits of paedophilia

I believe that paedophilia can be considered a sexual perversion with specific features. Perversions are characterised by a psychic withdrawal in which a sexual fantasy is central to the reaching of masturbatory pleasure. The basic fantasy and the way by which it is obtained varies according to the nature of the perversion (whether it be sado-masochism, exhibitionism, transvestism, fetishism, paedophilia, or other). The sexualised fantasy, already present in the early infancy of the future pervert, blocks the development of the healthy part of the personality luring it into the experience of addictive pleasure (De Masi, 2003[1999]).

In my opinion, paedophile perversion is sustained by a specific delusional nucleus, a *misconception* (Money-Kyrle, 1968), a pathological organisation of the internal world in which a highly idealised, venerated object treated like an idol takes the place of the parental figures.

This nucleus, split from the rest of the personality, appears to be the sole source of gratification and exerts a very strong power over the patient, orientating and colouring all aspects of his life. The split between the sexualised withdrawal and the rest of the personality is well described in the case presented by Socarides (1959). His patient, seriously traumatised from infancy, used to live two separate psychic lives. In one of them, which we will call A, the patient perceived himself as a kind person, capable of having relationships. When he was invaded by anxiety, he would enter psychic life B, in which the only aim was to sexually possess a young boy. During sexual activity, the partner was meant to remain immobile and not experience any pleasure. When the patient became B, he was quite unaware of the existence of A. The split between these two internal parts allowed him to carry on his paedophile activity without having to ever come into conflict with it.

Similarly, in the case reported by Glasser (1988), the patient had two ways of operating: the first was centred on the beauty of the adolescent, which led him to venerate the figure of the young boy; the second, instead, was totally sexualised and drove him to anal penetration of the young boy as a way of attaining a permanent orgasm.

My patient also presented an analogous split between idealising and sexualising aspects: the paedophile fantasy, however, did not intervene to sedate the anxiety but was part of a sophisticated and complex delusional construction. We may wonder what might have been the negative factors that pushed this patient towards an idealisation of the infantile world and to confer on the latter such a strongly delusional character. Some traumatic family patterns might have orientated him towards the world of paedophilia. His mother, who had stimulated his narcissistic expectations in early childhood, had subsequently betrayed him by falling in love with her son's playmate.

In analysis, the patient had progressively become aware that this maternal betrayal was at the basis of his homosexual orientation and his aversion to the female world, but he had also, unfortunately, devalued the male paternal world.

The sole world to survive and have become idealised was that of childhood–adolescence. This was the happy world of playfulness and imagination. The boys would immediately be distanced and lost when they grew up and started to express an interest in girls. Michele could not understand, literally, why, when attracted by female figures, boys would tend to remove themselves from the adolescent and exclusively male group.

I have several times emphasised the "romantic" element in Michele's paedophilia, which found its roots in his idealisation of the world of childhood. It was possible, in fact, to perceive some positive elements in his idealisation of this world, even though that same idealisation would entail an altered perception of psychic reality.

The most specifically perverse element of his paedophilia was strictly connected with his infantile sexualised withdrawal and included a sadomasochistic fantasy in which a dominated object would participate actively in the pleasure of the partner. One of the most frequent fantasies of that period was riding a horse, which in the end would collapse with exhaustion and surrender itself to his power and control. From this altruistic submission of the animal, which would exhaust itself on the orders of the master, the patient would receive enormous sensual pleasure

I thought it important, from a technical point of view, to keep separate and distinct the perverse and the idealising aspects, as I saw in the latter some relational elements that could be developed. As the analytic process progressed, the relation between the sexualising and the idealising parts has been modified to the advantage of the second. After the first period, characterised by the addictive, sadomasochistic excitement, we moved to the second, in which idealisation and fusional dependence on the world of childhood prevailed (this world being deployed partly in an anti-analytical mode). We eventually reached the third stage, in which the patient could face in a stable way his psychic and emotional worlds.

I believe that this transformation has been made possible by the fact that I have constantly placed myself alongside the patient when scrutinising his perverse fantasies, helping him, session after session, to distinguish between the healthy parts to be nurtured and the sexualised parts to be contained and transformed. In so doing, I was consistently preoccupied with analysing without let-up the confusional areas. The risk of being identified with an absent and confusing parent was always present and could become real as soon as my analytical responses were not discriminating enough.

In one session, for instance, Michele had brought the photo of an adolescent football team getting ready for a match. Two of the boys featured had their hands on their genitals. This was, for the patient, clear evidence that all adolescents masturbate each other. The polemical vehemence of the patient towards me (I was seen as an interlocutor denying his statement) had been so strong in that particular session that I had become unable to think. I trivialised the whole issue and ended by making the remark that the position of the boys' hands might have been completely casual. The following day, Michele came back even angrier. He attacked me by asserting that I had said that masturbating was normal, that all boys do it, and that I was like his mother, who invited him to masturbate (this was, in reality, what the mother would say when he was trying to explain to her the pleasure that he got from masturbation). I think that in this case the patient was right to attack me. I had not understood the problem of the previous session and I had behaved like a distracted and confusing mother. I had given him a trivialising answer, which he had taken as an invitation to masturbation, while he needed to perceive me as the parent who understands the experience of the child but does not support his sexualised excitement.

Long years of work have been necessary to allow the patient to escape the power of the sexualised area and to open himself to the emotional growth within the analytical relationship. When this happened, I realised the extent to which the sexualised withdrawal had stripped his mind, rendering the world of affective relationships very difficult to explore.

Because of the addictive quality of the sexualised nucleus, treatment of paedophile perversions turns out to be painstakingly long and hard. The main characteristic of this treatment is the initial distance between the two members of the analytic dyad. For, however much the analyst is prepared to understand the patient and to listen empathically to him, he will, to begin with, perceive the world of paedophilia as incomprehensible, disheartening, and distant.

In order that the hope of a possible transformation is not distorted by cynicism and by the obstinacy with which the patient defends his position, the analyst must maintain for a long time a balance and a sustained interest in the mysterious singularity of the paedophile world. We are not completely powerless in our dealing with paedophilia if we succeed in properly "understanding" it.

The outcome of this case suggests that, if analytically treated, some forms of paedophilia are open to therapeutic transformation. I must also emphasise, however, that, in Michele's case, the attraction towards the world of paedophilia was matched from the very beginning by the anxiety of becoming totally colonised and engulfed by it.

This element, which I considered positive from a prognostic point of view, may not be present in other cases of paedophile perversion.

In this chapter, I have tried to focus on the analytic relationship and on the evolution of the patient's paedophile nucleus. Therefore, I could not describe in detail the analytic work dedicated to the structure of his personality, to his anxieties akin to psychosis, and to his inclination towards sadomasochistic relations, all of which occupied the analytic transference for a long time. The patient's particular form of homosexuality, implying a total refusal and hatred for the female figure, was also dealt with extensively. However, paedophilia can develop in very different personality structures, as can be inferred from the literature on this subject, and as I have noticed in other cases brought to my attention.

CHAPTER ELEVEN

The enigma of transsexualism

"Ending sessions was very difficult for him. When he was told
that there were five minutes left before the end, he would pick
up Barbie and stroke her hair or would create images of women
by drawing them or constructing them with clay"

(From the therapy of Colin, in Coates & Moore, 1997, p. 297)

This chapter will explore the issue of whether or not common
characteristics are present in the various cases of transsexual
patients who have seen an analyst, and draws on the most
significant works in the psychoanalytic literature.

While the study of transsexualism has shed more light on the atypical experiences of child sexuality, the subject—due to its singular
nature—has long been marginal in psychoanalytic thought and is still
awaiting a more suitable clinical and theoretical collocation.

In fact, transsexualism has only become an object of systematic
study, carried out with great attention and rigour, in the past few
decades. Observations of small children who already show denial of
their gender identity at a very young age, often accompanied by a disturbed affective and relational life, have been particularly important.

This chapter reviews the main works on therapies of transsexual patients in the psychoanalytic literature; in no case with adults was it possible to modify their wish to change sex, while more positive outcomes were obtained with operated transsexual patients, who ask for help in coming to terms with their new state. The most successful therapeutic results are obtained with children because the structure of their personality is still malleable and susceptible to change.

Limentani (1979) postulates that transsexualism challenges the fundamental basis of the psychoanalytic edifice because it does not recognise the structuring role of the Oedipus complex. In fact, authors who deal with this theme have questioned Freud's assumption (1924d) that "anatomy is destiny".

In an attempt to formulate some hypotheses about the precocious and original conditions that further the formation of such a syndrome, I shall pay particular attention to the material involving transsexual children.

Transvestism and transsexualism: similarities and differences

Sexual identity, which is at the basis of personal identity, is one of the most important acquisitions to be made by children; suffice to think of how they refer to each other: "I'm a boy, you're a girl".

Male–female transsexuals, while anatomically male, believe they are women imprisoned in men's bodies; *vice versa*, women (female–male) transsexuals believe they are men imprisoned in women's bodies.

It is necessary to distinguish transvestism from transsexualism, even though there are various forms of transition between the two: in the former, the individual wears clothes of the opposite sex and derives enormous pleasure from doing so; in the latter, instead, the individual wishes to change sex. The transvestite wants to look like a woman; the transsexual wants to become a woman.

Sexual identity and gender identity

It has been known for some time that the subjective perception of sexual identity also depends on family and social influences and that sex does not determine gender.

For example, eyewitness accounts reported by early explorers in Central America describe how the fifth son born into native families that only had male children was destined to be female. To this end, from the beginning the baby boy was dressed as a girl and treated like one; as he grew, he acquired a feminine identity and behaved as a woman in his social relationships and social role.

Briggs (1986) describes the customs of people living in Labrador and in eastern Greenland in raising a child as a member of the opposite sex with the objective of reincarnating a dead person or of bringing up a future hunter if the family's children were all female. Some of these children maintain their transsexual identity for the rest of their lives; others, instead, abandon it as puberty sets in.

In the first years of life, children perceive themselves through the eyes of adults. Consequently, it is understandable that the first perception of identity depends on the image that parents send to their baby. Sexual identity, in particular, is attributed to the newborn by obstetricians and parents.

Stoller (1968) proposes distinguishing *sexual identity*, which refers to anatomy (the presence of a penis or a vagina), from *gender identity*, which concerns the subjective conviction of belonging to one or the other sex and which, consequently, might not correspond to sexual identity.

In one of his works, Stoller examined three children who, at a very early age, said they were female, dressed as girls, and had female attitudes. All three came from family nuclei dominated by an apprehensive, anxious mother who had no significant bond with her husband and who used the child as an object-self. The children were in constant physical contact with the mother, on whom they depended emotionally, and did not seem to be differentiated from her. Stoller postulates that in these cases the absence of the male figure creates an urge in the child to identify with the female figure.

The North American author claims that mothers of transsexuals have a girl in mind and psychologically treat their sons as though they were girls. As a general rule, in order to reach a gender identity in line with their anatomical sex, males have a rather more complex path to follow because they have to de-identify themselves from the primitive fusion with the mother and achieve a separate identity. For this reason, disorders of sexual identity are more frequent in males than in females.

Core gender identity, derived from the attribution of sex on the part of the environment, is established, according to Stoller (1964), within the first three years of life and is destined to be preserved during development, whereas gender identity is consolidated by the end of adolescence.

Ovesey and Person (1973) present a different thesis from that put forward by Stoller. Using the concept of separation anxiety, the two American authors propose a psychodynamic explanation of trans-sexualism as the result of a defensive reaction to anxiety: the threat of fragmentation and annihilation would push the child towards a fantasy of symbiotic fusion with the mother. These would be highly anxious children who are unable to separate from the mother and who identify with her in an attempt to deny separation. Therefore, they are emotionally withdrawn, asexual children with a schizoid type of func-tioning. The mothers of the transsexuals described by Ovesey and Person are conscientious but cold women, indifferent to the vital needs of their children.

Following the same line of thought, other authors (Coates, Fried-man, & Wolfe, 1991) postulate that transsexualism is a strategy used by the child to face his separation anxiety. The children in question develop what Coates (2006) equates to a kind of reparative fantasy, that is, a female identification with the mother. Genetic factors, too, play a role in pushing the child towards the transsexual solution.

Primary and secondary transsexualism

Ovesey and Person (1973) also make another important distinction: between *primary* and *secondary transsexualism*. They are convinced that an individual is not always a transsexual at birth, but often becomes one. Primary transsexualism includes subjects that present an ambiguous core gender from early infancy. Secondary transsexuals, instead, are individuals who have been homosexual or practised cross-dressing for years before becoming transsexuals: at a certain point it was no longer enough for them just to wear women's clothes, they had to change sex.

Primary transsexualism does not imply a homosexual organisation of the personality. Fantasying about being a girl or young woman and wearing female clothes provides warmth and pleasure; this type of transsexual begins by dressing up in female clothes when very young and, until a certain age, tries to combat the fantasy of being a woman. After adolescence, the attempt to establish gender identity according to anatomical sex is abandoned and he lives as "a woman in spirit inside a man's body".

In contrast, secondary transsexualism implies a transition from homosexuality or from transvestism or from both states to transsexualism.

The distinction between transvestism and transsexualism is not always linear. Transvestites are aroused by wearing female clothes, but conserve their own gender identity. Often recourse to transvestism is an impulsive way of behaving, especially when the individual wants to shake off a state of mental suffering. Some adult transsexuals remember that when they were small they used to dress up in their mother's or sister's clothes or underwear and feeling strangely attracted by the touch of the soft female undergarments.

Clinical cases

I would now like to present a number of clinical cases of patients who have come directly or indirectly under my observation.

It is well known that the transsexual patient finds it difficult to accept the idea of coming to a proper analysis: there is a risk, for him, that a lifetime dream that can now be realised thanks to new surgical techniques will be destroyed. The patient does not trust the analyst, since he believes that the analyst's sole objective is to persuade him to renounce the operation. This is why so very few cases are described in analytic literature.

However, it would seem to me that the material, even if it cannot be held to be a true therapy, can be useful for providing elements for further reflection on the complex issues of the problem.

Renato

Below, I report two interviews with a child who can be considered a case of primary transsexualism.

Renato is six years old and attends the first year of primary school. His teachers have told his parents that he has considerable difficulty in paying attention and concentrating.[14]

His parents are about thirty years old; his mother is an employee and his father is a goldsmith. They say that Renato, ever since he was tiny, was attracted to girls' games and the company of girls; he said he loved them and did not know whether he wanted to be a boy or a girl. The child has always had a privileged relationship with his mother, also because his father was generally always at work or busy with his hobby (he plays in a small band).

Renato is afraid of the dark to such an extent that he cannot go to the bathroom by himself; it is very unlikely that he will ask to go outside because a mere nothing frightens him. He plays almost all the time with "Winx" fairies and loves to watch cartoons on television. At home he cannot finish even the simplest of tasks, like taking off his shoes, for example, or washing his hands, because he is always distracted by imagining games to play with the dolls.

In the first interview he said he was no good at school because he likes to play with girls' things, dolls, and his friends make fun of him for this. He gets distracted, thinks about other things, and wastes time because he senses they are laughing at him even if their desks are quite far from his.

He adds that he does not like playing very much . . . he likes to stay at home all day and watch television; his mother lets him watch cartoons and, sometimes, she even lets him eat in front of the TV! He never has school friends home to play. When the analyst asks him to talk about his father he says, "My father is handsome, he has a beautiful face, because I like people if they have beautiful faces . . . He's also strong because sometimes he is strong enough to break your bones, when he hits me, I feel that . . . But I don't speak to my father, I've never spoken to him . . . I don't really like boys . . . I can talk to girls, I'm calmer . . . my father, when he gets cross, he gets terribly angry . . . I've got a friend who comes to my house to play. I like playing with her with the Barbies . . . and then, you know, my father works for himself, he comes home late and then, some evenings, he goes to play with his band . . . He's never here."

He adds that he is afraid of boys and also of the dark: ". . . you see, I see my favourite toys start to change as soon as the light grows dim, and it looks as though they are turning into something strange."

At this point, it seems as though Renato wants to draw. First he plans to draw his mother, who never wears a skirt, but then he wants to draw the

Barbie he is holding. He says he will put her in a flower and she will be a princess (Figure 1).

In the second interview, Renato comes into the room, takes a Barbie and sits down silently. Then he says that they make fun of him at school because he plays with dolls; he likes the "Winx" a lot, and really wants to be Stella. Renato adds, "You know, I want to tell you something else: I have bad dreams at night. I dreamt that a wolf was coming, he wanted to eat me up but killed me first with a knife. I'm frightened of nastiness and my schoolmates are always playing games in which they are pushing and shouting . . . they aren't calm, they are bad, they are bossy . . . and I don't play with them. I've got something else to tell you: I see people who turn into wolves . . . except for mum and dad and Alessia and Niccolò . . . and my grandparents, and you."

He draws his family (Figure 2). He gets distracted and starts talking about how frightened he is of the wolf in *Little Red Riding Hood* and of the one in the *Three Little Pigs*.

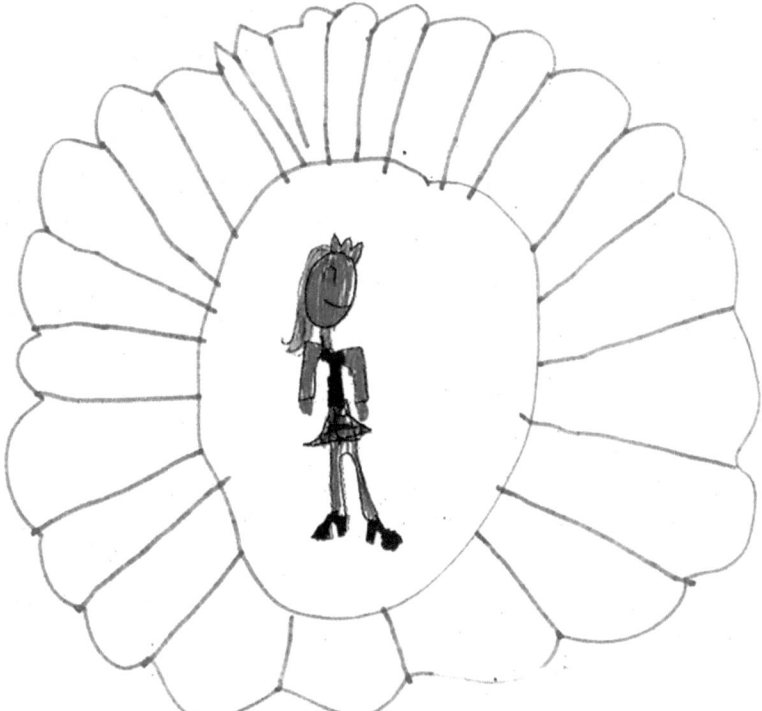

Figure 1.   Renato's drawing of his Barbie as a princess in a flower.

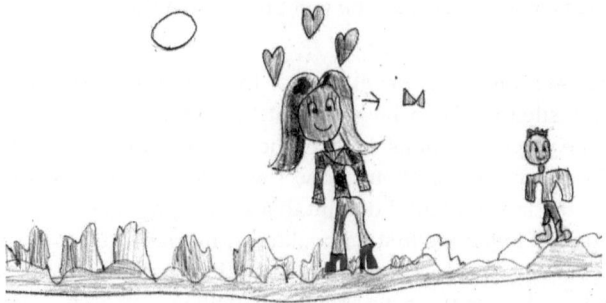

Figure 2.   Renato's drawing of his family.

"And I also think of illness: I'm afraid of getting sick because some illnesses get inside you and ruin your skin; your skin goes all wrinkled. I'm frightened of my face getting ugly."

Renato certainly seems to be a case of primary transsexualism, a child moving precociously towards a gender identity in clear contrast with his anatomical sex.

The most striking thing is that Renato lives most of his day immersed in dreams and an enchanted world. The fantasies with which he transforms his perceptions are not always pleasurable; they are also bearers of anxiety and death and persecution. Part of his persecutory anxiety is projected on to his male schoolmates who, because of their vivacity, are experienced as dangerous. It is likely that his desire to live in a female world is also nourished by his anxiety towards the male world, felt as strongly aggressive and persecutory (as in the dream about the wolf). This leads to an idealising of the female world that stimulates the wish that he himself may become a woman.

But what type of woman does Renato have in mind? The woman in his drawing is a queen who lives an enchanted life in the corolla of a daisy.

From what his parents say, it can be inferred that Renato experienced a privileged relationship with his mother in the first months of his life and that his father is emotionally distant. In fact, in the drawing of his family, the figure of the father is totally absent. The child drew first himself and then his mother. It is interesting to note that when he represents himself within the family, he draws himself as a male, while in his lonely imagination he is a female. Renato did not finish the drawing because when he began to draw the female figure he became totally absorbed by his imaginary world focused on the woman. More than the mother, this refers to the female figure *per se*, or even to the "Winx" fairies, powerful and capable of experiencing exciting emotions. It must also be noted how he expresses himself about his father: he speaks of him in a very adult way as though he really was an adolescent, both attracted to the strength and figure of the man and fearful of it.

He appreciates his father's beauty, and the smoothness of his skin, which already seems to have reached the level of a fetish for him. However, he feels that this idealised surface can easily be ruined (even illness or age can wrinkle his skin) and so the anxiety returns with all its strength.

This child resembles a case described by Chiland (2000). Antoine, too, had drawn a blonde princess, very different from his real mother with dark hair. Later, a dark and dangerous female figure would appear next to this idealised woman.

From transvestism to transsexualism

In the attempt to make a connection between the various symptomatologies that rotate around the issue of transsexualism, Di Ceglie (1998) puts forward a proposal to use the term "atypical gender identity organisation" (AGIO) for a vast phenomenology that ranges from gender identity at odds with sexual identity, to the way of dressing, to the use of toys and role plays, and to anatomical dysphoria (intense revulsion for the sexed body). The author points out that the desire to change sex does not always constitute a system of unshakable beliefs, as described by Stoller. The atypical organisations that develop very early can be tenacious, while others that form later and are linked to emotional traumas can be transformed more easily. Only systematic exploration provides the answer as to how rigid this type of organisation is.

I shall now present three clinical cases of adults that show a significant passage from playing the female role (transvestism) to seeking a true sex change. The first account describes a case of transvestism.

Ivano

Ivano asks for a consultation on the advice of his wife, the only person to know that "I like to dress as a woman". I report only the initial interviews of this patient because, after the first exploratory discussions, he decided to put off the start of analysis, giving family motives and lack of time as reasons.

Ivano's father, the founder and director of a big successful business, is a myth for the family while his mother, who busied herself with the house and children, is an anxious person subject to cyclical depression. Ivano is the last-born of four children: two boys and two girls. The first-born sister took care of him and was his real mother. Ivano is married and is thirty-two years old. He is very keen on the theatre and film and writes amateur film scripts. A recurrent theme in his tales is the story of weak, sensitive women whose life has been marked by destiny. Knowing his particular passions, Ivano's wife gives him female underwear that he wears in their sexual relations. If she openly praises his clothing, his arousal increases notably. He often masturbates in front of the mirror imagining stories in which he, dressed as a woman, pretends to be a dressmaker who receives a man at home. This clean-shaven effeminate young man makes appreciative comments about him and tells him not to pretend because it is obvious that he is a man who likes to dress as a woman. The two begin to touch each other and masturbate. The most exciting element for him is the tactile sensation of women's underwear on his skin. If he could, Ivano would be reborn as a woman. He began dressing up when he was six years old, putting on his two older sisters' underwear. He nurtured his inclination "to be in contact with women" by attending a dressmaking course and then as a nurse in the Red Cross. He was a sad and lonely child in infancy and adolescence: he suffered from intense homesickness every time he left home, even for brief periods.

Now his wife is expecting their first child. Ivano thinks that the birth of this child will force him to give up his fantasy of wanting to be a woman and dressing up. He cannot conceive of being a father that plays with these things; what example would he be for his son? At the same time he says, "If it was up to me, I would go far away, to a country where no one knows me, so that I could become a woman."

Ivano speaks of his passion for transvestite porn mags: he is attracted to photos of men dressed as women that bear a resemblance to him; he recalls his childhood when he went to the nuns' nursery school and loved touching the material of their habits. When he thinks of his wife's pregnancy, he hopes it will be a little girl. He would send her to a convent of nuns but, he adds, he would forego having a son or daughter if he himself could enter a convent and become a novitiate. He has always liked the idea of being able to wear a uniform and live a life ordered by rules. When he was doing the nursing course, he was fascinated by the idea of living in a convent. The pleasure, he says, derives not so much from the sacrifice in itself as in losing one's freedom and being subject to a superior. Ivano imagines arriving at the convent: a nun will welcome him, take away his clothes and give him the garments of the order. He will have to bind his chest to hide his breasts. He sees himself as a simple nun, not as a mother superior because a position of command would remove the pleasure of being subjected and suffering punishment. In this fantasy, he breaks one of the rigid monastic rules. So he imagines he has to be punished: he has to do the hard work, remain kneeling for hours on end or remain in silence. All these fantasies are played out on the backdrop of his childhood nursery school. That place was sad, but he was happy when he could speak to a girl cousin his own age. He remembers that the most important thing about his childhood was living much of his free time in female groups. He spent the holidays with a sister and her friends; the girls were self-assured and pretty; they spoke nicely but seemed unreachable.

Talking about the family business that he works in, he also thinks back to the emotional climate in which he grew up. A state of undifferentiation reigned in his family, a calm that prevented any expression of emotion. Everything was subordinated to his father's success in industry. One's duty was to be good and not create any trouble. Even now Ivano has not told anyone he wants to begin analysis. The flat and impersonal atmosphere of his life is repeated in his film scripts. They narrate stories of women who work on the assembly line or who live out a banal existence that is then suddenly changed by fate and meeting the love of their lives.

*   *   *

Many of Ivano's fantasies refer directly back to his childhood, to his time at nursery school, and to his female companions (the nuns, his sisters, and their friends). His wish to be a woman is accompanied by masochistic fantasies, by an attraction for mortifying the self, by the claustrophilia of convent life, and by submission to hierarchy. Even if the desire to become a woman involves a masochistic element (it is, in any case, a self-castration), Ovesey and Person (1973) state that it is not infrequent for the transvestite to have specific masochistic fantasies.

Ivano's story makes one think that something vital has been lost in his earliest infancy. If his father was distant and his brother emotionally inconsistent, was it not natural for him to identify with his sister, who was perhaps the only vitally alive person? Ivano takes inside himself not only his sister's vital character but also wants "to be" like his sister; he would willingly exchange his person with hers, with her appearance and her identity.

In a transvestite patient such as Ivano, the male body is not hated as it is by a transsexual. He does not really want to change physical identity; in his fantasy, it is essential to be able to personify a female role, which is also fundamental for reaching sexual arousal.

The request for an analytic consultation seems to me to be connected to the anxiety triggered by the conflict between his fantasy of being a woman and the push to take on the role of father for the approaching birth of his first child.

Mario

Mario began analysis (four sessions a week) at the age of thirty.[15] He confesses that he is overwhelmed by panic when he is involved in an emotional or sexual relationship with a possible girlfriend: in that moment he has to imagine the presence of other male or female partners in the act; without this stimulus of promiscuity, his desire evaporates.

Virtual sex is more important for him than real sex; it is the only thing that triggers his desire. He often makes use of fee-paying hardcore phone chats or trawls pornographic websites. One of his passions is to collect photos and personal information about the most beautiful women in the world: he has at least a hundred for each one.

In his case, too, the erotic withdrawal began in childhood. He says that his mother was very worried about his health and kept him in the big parental bed in place of his father. Since he was small he has been attracted by female bodies, as though there is something extraordinarily exciting in women that must be grasped and taken for himself. He often had erotic dreams about his mother or spied on her, when he could, to see her half naked in the bath. When little, he remembers often wearing her underwear to excite himself in front of the mirror. Looking at images of nude women today still exercises a hypnotic fascination over him.

When he is gripped by anxiety he has an uncontrollable need for the sexual female world; he has to activate hard-porn phone calls or run to the computer and immediately immerse himself in pornographic sites. Using the Internet not only serves to placate his anxiety, it is also a path that, having been travelled repeatedly, tends to alter his identity. From a certain moment onwards, Mario does not just look or chat on the Internet, he begins to want to become a woman who arouses men. He begins to dress, puts on make-up, and then rushes down into the street. In these moments, Mario is totally identified with the desired object and becomes that vast beauty that so attracts him. He brings his photos in female dress to the analyst and also arrives at the sessions made up like a woman with the aim of finding confirmation of the successful transformation that has occurred.

* * *

I have described this patient to show that, even in the case of transvestism, the initial nucleus of the eroticised withdrawal begins in childhood. Unlike Ivano, in Mario's case the pleasure in being a woman is taking an increasingly stronger hold over him and it is not easy to foresee the outcome. For example, it can be hypothesised that Mario will not stop at being a transvestite, but, in the absence of any containing therapy, will press onwards until the moment he asks for a surgical transformation.

Fausto

I have recently supervised the psychotherapy of a young transsexual who had already planned to have, and had made the necessary arrangements for, the surgical intervention with a specialised centre.

* * *

Fausto[16] is nineteen years old and is an intelligent, good-looking student. He left school during his last year of high school. This is how he presented himself at the first consultation: "My problem, in a few short words, is that I am a woman—that's it. Despite all appearances, I am a woman. Unfortunately, no one, first of all no one in my family, has ever understood this. Since I was small I have always played with girls and I liked their games. We laughed together . . . I know quite certainly that no analysis in the world will change me. I feel good only when I put on my mother's clothes. If I dress as a woman, I am reborn; I feel better, I live another life, it has a physical effect on me, it comforts me. As for my body, I'd like it to take on female aspects; I take hormones, even though I know they can be dangerous."

Fausto continues and makes extremely pertinent comments that denote pharmaceutical and endocrinological competence. He prescribes the hormones himself thanks to a prescription he has falsified: "Look doctor, I'm not mad, I do it because I know I'm right, I know that it's the only way to save myself. I cannot and am unable to live life as a male."

In his family, he lives in an atmosphere of incomprehension and rigidity, which was further exasperated after his explicit declaration of wanting to be a woman. He was also planning to operate on himself and had already bought all the necessary equipment—surgical knives, disinfectant, and so on. At a certain point, the patient exclaims, "You don't want to send me to hospital do you? Everyone wants to send me to hospital because I'm different." And he goes on to ask, "All the doctors I've been to have given me medicines; what will you give me?"

In the second consultation, he took up the tale of his childhood. When young he had had difficulty playing with children of the same age. He did not identify with his father or play "boys' games". His father's car soon ceased to interest him. Instead, he remembers putting on his mother's high heels and making a terrible noise with them around the house. He was excellent at school. He was also very musical but, after winning a prize for the violin, had given up music because he had noticed that having a gifted son gave his parents a lot of satisfaction.

He often felt enclosed in a "black hole" and stayed for hours under the table. He was sad and everything around him was gloomy. He was happy only when he met twin girls who lived in the same building.

He spied on them; he peeped through the keyhole when they changed their clothes; he was fascinated by their smooth bodies, lacking the "appendage" of a penis.

He brought a dream to the third consultation:

> "I dreamt I was putting on a pair of tights, the transparent kind. The other day I tried them, they were my mother's . . . in the dream I only had one stocking, a single leg. I didn't have the other one. How on earth could I have gone out like that? So my father got me the other one . . . so I put it on . . . and I felt better . . ."

He associates the dream to the fact that the day before his father, most unusually, had seemed to be more accepting of his plan to become a woman. From what emerges of the patient's story, his father is a really dominating and aggressive person. His intolerance towards his son reaches heights of worrying violence, so that this surprisingly conciliatory attitude is a rare event.

* * *

In the real world, Fausto's father obstructs his son's desire. The dream shows that although Fausto declares to the analyst that he is certain about his choice, inside himself he is not so certain about whether to wear one or two stockings. In the dream, he projects his anxiety about the decision on to his father (and, in the transference, on to the analyst), who provides the solution.

The contents of the dream are also connected to the relationship that Fausto has with the surgical department of the hospital, where he has planned to have the operation. The psychologist of the centre is insisting that he is operated on quickly.

I would like to add a few words about the relationship between the patient and the maternal figure. His mother is a closed woman, hard and rigid, who had devoted herself exclusively to her work when her son was young, often being away from home. The patient was entrusted to his grandmother, who treated him severely: there was constant conflict between the two of them. Fausto remembers that he used to provoke her until she lost her temper. Once, he had shut her outside on the balcony, where she had stayed for a long time in the cold, subsequently falling ill with bronchitis.

Fausto is convinced that his aggressive, metallic mother has never loved him. Instead, he recalls with immense pleasure the happy moments spent playing with the twins of his own age. It seems that, persecuted by a sense of profound non-existence, the prisoner of a "black hole", Fausto had believed he could escape it with a butterfly's wings, transforming himself into a female figure, the pleasing and exciting vision of the twins.

Problems linked with his transsexual wish followed by arguments with his father, and by the difficulty of returning to high school, emerged in the sessions.

During the first year, Fausto returned to school and to relating with his classmates. While his desire to undergo the surgical operation lessened, he fell in love platonically with a boy of his own age at school. Before therapy, he had attempted a number of homosexual encounters, but had immediately broken them off because he wanted to be treated like a woman and not like a man. At present, he has a stable companion with whom he has a good affective relationship.

As for his transsexual issues, this patient showed a relatively rapid development. It was necessary to listen, grasp, and understand the world of this young man in much greater depth, especially his polemical isolation within his family. It was important to keep in mind that the desire to become a woman was a powerful defence against infantile depression and that it was not possible to question it at the beginning of treatment.

*   *   *

Fausto said, "When I was little, my parents weren't there, or, if they were there,; they didn't treat me so that I could understand that I was their son; they were always worried, semi-depressed. I remember a sort of black shell that enveloped me and that made a nest for me under the kitchen table; I stayed there for hours, alone, like that."

*   *   *

After six months of therapy, he declared that he no longer wanted to change sex, that it would have been an incredibly stupid thing to do, and that now he knew he wanted to stay being a man. I think it is important to note that the therapist remained vigilant but neutral and did not—unlike his father in the dream—provide him with the other stocking.

Another factor that bolstered his wish to change derived from what the patient experienced in the meetings with the psychologist of the hospital where he would have had the operation; this person seemed to be pushing him towards the operation, inciting him to be more courageous.

In contrast, the therapeutic work offered him the time and space necessary for taking a decision. Helping to demythologise the sex change as a way of obtaining an impossible happiness helped Fausto to overcome the conflict with his family and to get closer to people of his own age.

It is interesting to observe how Fausto finds himself having to deal with the identity void that follows from the loss of his illusory personality when he abandoned his plan for a sex change. This is how he communicates his change of heart to the therapist.

* * *

"I've not said anything to my parents yet, but I wanted to tell you, I've decided not to go ahead with the treatment at the hospital . . . it happened after thinking about it all again this weekend, when I also saw Giorgio, but when I was also alone; I thought that I don't feel like doing the operation any more and that everything I do is something pathological, not normal . . . you can't believe how hard it is. I also reread Semi [Antonio Semi, *Trattato di Psicoanalisi*, 1997], also because we spoke here about being psychotic, that I would pathologically identify myself with a female figure, and I found the word transvestism in Semi. I recognised myself, that's me. It always happens like that with me, to go from idealisation to idealisation, putting myself in the place of the subject that I idealise . . . it was like that being a woman. I'm afraid that this stage will pass, that I will go back to feeling myself such . . . a woman; I feel totally sick. I will go and explain to the endocrinologist that I am not a woman and I have decided not to have the operation. I realise I have been depressed ever since I was little. It's as though I realised that I have been living in a non-real world, that I am not real and now I feel sort of discouraged about everything. In actual fact, I'm really sad, my parents don't understand my problem. I hope this conviction stays with me and I will speak to the doctor at the hospital . . . it's the transvestism that Semi talks of; I identified with something outside me."

* * *

The fact that this patient changed his idea quite rapidly poses some questions of a diagnostic nature. Can we consider Fausto to be a "true" transsexual, or is a hysterical component present in his wish to change sex?

Granted, in childhood he did not like playing boys' games, he enjoyed putting on his mother's high heels, and was very isolated in respect of his peers, but as a small boy he never manifested any desire to become a woman. He only conceived the fantasy of the operation in adolescence, after acknowledging that he was homosexual. Even if he proclaimed in words his wish to be operated on and had made contact with the surgical department of the hospital, deeper down he seemed quite doubtful about it all. The dream of the stockings shows that Fausto does not express an absolutely certain desire for bodily transformation but was waiting for encouragement from his father.

It is probable that the understanding, empathic attitude of the therapist and, later, better acceptance by his parents diminished the polemical and provocative potential inherent in the request to change sex. It would seem that in the dynamics of this case, the prevailing feelings were both conscious and unconscious hatred for his parents, devoid of any generating function, and that his rebirth as a woman would have been a manic triumph against them (Oppenheimer, 1991).

Similar cases of transitory transsexual vocations exist that have to be distinguished from true transsexualism.

Therapies for transsexuals

The therapeutic path for transsexuals is very complex. Chiland (1998) says that when one attempts to discuss problems inherent to the patients' project for bodily transformation, they become irritated and abandon therapy. Except for one case described by Ruth Stein (1995), there are no adult patients in the analytic literature who decide on a therapeutic course as an alternative to the surgical intervention. Indeed, before the operation, the prospect of psychological therapy is seen as counter to the only solution to the problem—surgery—for which they have fought for years.

Only after the operation do these patients sometimes ask for psychological help because the bodily transformation did not bring the longed-for serenity while problems, uncertainties, and personal discomfort emerge that the new state has not dispelled.

The mass media generally proffer superficial and banal information that makes a sex change seem a relatively easy undertaking. Even the medical–surgical organisation, proud of its success stories, tends to encourage body transformation; the message spread by the actors of today's technological omnipotence is that anything is possible and in a very short time.

However, it is recorded that not all patients who have undergone surgery are satisfied with having finally achieved what they had long desired; sometimes they are disappointed or very angry, to the point, in some cases, of thinking of suicide.

Hakeem (2007) reports the many years of experience of the Portman Clinic (London) in providing group therapy for suffering operated patients with the aim of helping them deal with depression and prevent the risk of suicide.

However, even in the best cases, the problems do not disappear after the operation. The operated male to female transsexual has to resolve complex bodily issues, starting with the vagina implant that has to be constantly canalised. With female to male transsexuals, there is the grafting of a penis that will never perform its sexual or reproductive functions.

Moreover, complex emotional, psychological, and sexual issues especially emerge after the operation, as can be seen in the case described in two different moments by Quinodoz (1998, 2002). A critical moment was reached in the analytic story of her patient, who had been surgically changed to a woman before the start of analysis, when she started to become aware that she could not transform her past in a way that convinced her that she had always been a woman. It took much difficult analytic work for the patient to accept that she would have to live with an ambiguous identity; she could not consider herself a woman in the past, and neither could she think of herself as one in the future: for example, she would never even be able to have, like all women, the experience of the menopause. As the only identity possible, she had to accept that she was transsexual.

This case clearly shows that gender identity is a psychic and emotional construction that takes shape from the first relational experiences in infancy and that cannot be achieved only through bodily transformation. The surgical operation changes the anatomical aspect but is obviously not capable of establishing, *a posteriori*, the internalised emotional relations that are profoundly linked to the body's functions and that acquire great symbolic and identity value. Even simple somatic manifestations (for example, menstruation) have an imaginative and affective significance that the operated transsexual will never be able to feel as an intrinsic part of him.

The most positive therapeutic results in the case of transsexual patients can be found in precocious treatments during childhood. Two are described in the literature. One case of primary transsexualism in therapy is described by Coates and Moore (1997).

* * *

Three-and-a-half-year-old Colin had begun to say he was a girl and to put on his mother's clothes. He loved women's jewellery, he played with Barbie dolls, and loved the heroines in television cartoons. He was afraid of boys and of women with "angry eyes". He showed an acute sensitivity for colours and clothes. He was very attentive with his mother and constantly worried about her state of mind.

His mother was not very happy to have conceived him and his father had abandoned them soon after his birth. The greatest trauma occurred shortly after he was two years old, when his mother, pregnant again and certain she was going to have a little girl, had miscarried, and immediately following that her character changed: she became tense and worried and, in particular, became distant towards Colin, treating him harshly whenever he attempted to get close to her.

* * *

The authors postulate that the mother's mourning for the loss of her baby girl may have pushed Colin to want to be female. His fantasy was to be able to rediscover, as a girl, the contact he had lost with his mother. With her angry explosions, she had traumatised her son, who from that moment had begun to be frightened of women with angry eyes. Colin, too, like the child Renato discussed above, drew his family without the father figure.

At the end of therapy, Colin no longer wanted to become a girl; he had developed the knack of playing with boys his own age and of using his fantasy in a creative way. It must be added that his mother, too, had also decided to go into analysis in the same period and this can only have helped her child's developmental progress.

Another successful child therapy is described by Busch de Ahumada (2003). In this case, too, the child Jaime's behaviour was typical.

* * *

The fourth son of many siblings, he was at his happiest when he was able to be part of the group of his sisters. He loved to play with Barbie dolls and spent hours dressing them up and covering them with necklaces and rings. He was particularly attracted to long female hair, which he tried to touch and stroke constantly. Naturally, he did not play with children of his own age or with his brothers, and when he was at nursery school he stayed huddled on his own in a corner. Here, too, there was a history of maternal depression: after an abortion, which had occurred when he was one, his mother had left the family.

* * *

The author describes the psychic catastrophe that had struck the little boy and that had triggered an autistic withdrawal, fostering an illusional attempt to blend with the maternal body as a way of filling the emotional void.

Anatomy is not destiny

Study of the transsexual phenomenon has made clear that the construction of gender identity has complex transgenerational, psychic, and biological origins, which continuously influence each other and interact. Although, in some cases, it is abundantly clear that maternal wishes push the child towards a female identity, in other cases the parents are absent or uninterested in him.

Some authors almost fully agree in claiming that there is a narcissistic pathology at the root of transsexualism in which the patient, with a very low opinion of himself, tries to make manic-type repairs (Chiland, 2004; Oppenheimer, 1991).

The environmental components and the specific dynamics vary, however, from case to case.

Complex emotional issues that are still to be clarified are at the base of the desire of some girls who want to become boys, a rarer phenomenon compared to boys and one that appears later. The girl's desire to be a boy can derive from a debased view of the maternal figure, perceived as weak, resulting in no identification with her.

One of my patients of this type, who had reached adulthood with an under-defined gender identity, had always dressed as a boy since she was little, and obstinately refused to wear skirts. On growing up, she had dithered for a long time between homosexuality and hetero-sexuality, finally opting, during analysis, for the latter.

The refusal to identify with her mother is the decisive element in the case of the young woman described by Di Ceglie (1998).

* * *

Jennifer was seventeen when seen for the first time. She seemed a borderline personality with depressive episodes. She is the third child and has two older sisters; her mother, recently passed away, had also suffered from depressive episodes, one of which had occurred after the abortion of a male foetus that had shortly preceded Jennifer's birth. Her father was a violent man who continually hit her mother. Greatly embarrassed, Jennifer confessed that she identified with her father rather than her mother. She had always loved her mother and always dreamt of being able to do something extraordinary to make her happy. Perhaps her desire to be a man strong enough to defend her mother derives from this.

The psychotherapy allowed Jennifer to reconstruct her childhood story and to improve her social relations, but it did not succeed in transforming her transsexuality, which had probably manifested itself too precociously and had been reinforced by traumatic family experiences.

* * *

Di Ceglie (2000), again, relates the case of Christine.

* * *

Twelve-year-old Christine had been considered and treated as a boy by her mother, who did not deny her daughter's anatomical female conformation but declared that, on growing, she would become a boy. Despite growing up in these conditions, Christine does not present a consolidated gender identity disorder; she remembers she felt confused by her mother's ideas as a little girl, but, once puberty arrived, she felt herself definitely female.

* * *

According to the author, this clinical case demonstrates that environmental conditions alone are often not enough to determine gender identity.

Primary depression

The transsexual problem seems to be the expression of a complex set of circumstances that goes beyond the choice of gender identity. As is clearly seen in the analytic literature and in the clinical cases reported, children with primary transsexualism suffer from anxiety that seriously limits their capacity for growth and relations; they are not able to develop the vital aggressiveness that allows contact with reality and a relationship of exchanges with contemporaries. In some children, a compensatory withdrawal into a world of fantasy, dissociated from real relations, is evident. Older patients often remember a sad, lonely childhood, at times illuminated by female presences, of the same age or older sisters, without any significant male figure.

In the attempt to understand the original conditions that can foster the transsexual disorder, Oppenheimer (1991) identifies a disturbed relationship with the mother that prevents the development of a primary identity and that also has an impact on sexual gender.

In particular, the child destined to become transsexual already lives in a fantasy world that corresponds to a dissociated reality, and one of the characters in the fantasy (generally an idealised female figure) will be used as an image for a pathological identification. This point is strongly emphasised also by Chiland (2009), who believes that the transsexual child does not identify with the real mother, but with a highly idealised figure. What is more, alongside the idealised female figure there is another, but dangerous and threatening, by whom the child feels persecuted.

It can be said that the M–F transsexual's desire is upheld by a massive projective identification, a fantasy of appropriating the body and genitals of an idealised female figure who serves as a defence against an underlying primary depression. I use the term projective identification, following Klein's paper (1946), as a mechanism present in psychotic patients who, in appropriating brilliant aspects of an object in fantasy, succeed in changing their own identity.

This fantasy of changing identity, which has the strength of a delusional idea and which negates bodily and psychic reality, prevents the child from reaching a sexual identity corresponding to his anatomy.

The fantasy of appropriating female genitals is clearly expressed in the material that an American colleague, Vaia Tsolas, brought to the International Congress of Psychoanalysis in Berlin (2007).

* * *

A male transvestite, about fifty years old, suffering from character disorders and panic attacks, while waiting for the surgical operation, dreams of finding himself in a deserted house, very dirty and dilapidated, in which there is a wardrobe containing a jewellery box. He opens it, takes the jewels and puts them in his pocket, but in that moment his mother arrives and looks disapprovingly at him. Outside the window he sees children playing and he is worried because he might hurt them on falling.

* * *

Clearly, the dream stages the theft of identity: the patient steals the female identity and then naturally feels persecuted by the object that was stolen (the mother). The basic unhappiness and depression (the very dirty house) do not, though, miraculously disappear on stealing the identity, even if it is full of promises and symbolic significances.

The transsexual seems to want to take the woman's exciting attributes, her bodily appearance; the urgency of his desire is mainly focused on the pleasure in possessing parts of the female body, above all the breast and the smooth, hairless skin, and in wearing her soft clothes. It is a sensory pleasure in which the body is hyper-invested in a compensatory withdrawal (Chiland's "illness of narcissism"). In other words, in the transsexual's mind, the wish to change sex is upheld by the promise of achieving a happiness that has always been denied him.

Regarding this, Chiland (2005[1997]) states that the desire for maternity does not emerge in these patients: the possibility of procreating is not part of the dynamics of a transsexual's wishes.[17] Similarly, sexual desire would remain in the background. The plastic surgery most often requested by M–F transsexuals is to have breasts. According to Chiland, this would explain why the request for a surgical transformation is, in the first place, directed towards the desire of being recognised as female, and only secondly towards the desire for satisfying relationships with the other sex.

If we consider the cases of children with gender identity disorders documented in the literature, we can say that the nucleus of their sufferings is connected to a precocious psychic catastrophe (Busch de Ahumada, 2003).

Coates (2006) upholds that transsexualism is an intrapsychic solution for coming to terms with a very profound anxiety that leads to the construction of a false self. Commenting on the work of Coates, Spensley (2006) underlines the fact that, as well as the false self, a delusional self is structured that was constructed in fantasy.

Oppenheimer (1991), too, is convinced that transsexualism is structured in accordance with the two periods of psychosis (Freud, 1924e): withdrawal from reality (the reality of sex) and the creation of a neo-reality (the female body and the role of gender). The author assimilates the transsexual's neo-reality to the reconstructive work of delusion (Freud, 1911c). Argentieri (2006) points out that a clear contrast exists in transsexuals and transvestites between the relatively well-functioning part of the ego that is in contact with reality and the delusion involving sexual gender. This is why the author believes that these clinical cases, which are articulated in many forms of transition, all present the defensive mechanism of perversion, or, in other words, the denial and consequent unequal structural split of the ego, as indicated by Freud (1927e) for fetishism.

At this point, on the basis of the convergences mentioned above, we can formulate the hypothesis that transsexualism is the outcome of a state of infantile suffering that has involved the construction of defences that, as well as distorting emotional development, have interfered with the process of acquiring gender identity.

The psychodynamic sequence could be:

- a depressive void in the child (a serious primary depression) with persecutory anxiety regarding male aggression;
- a psychotic construction of a manic type obtained through projective identification with a brilliant female object, a transformation that promises happiness. In the case of F–M transsexualism, the idealised object that upholds the delusional desire is a male.

As highlighted by many authors, transsexualism would, therefore, be a blend of anxiety and narcissistic defences that do not remain as such, but that become structured in a delusional transformation of identity.

At this point, it is important to take up an observation made by Di Ceglie (1998, 2009) who, in hypothesising a close connection between emotional trauma and the development of the fantasy of bodily change, maintains that the earlier the trauma, the more rigid and unalterable the transsexual organisation.

The fact that at the basis of some forms of primary transsexualism lies a depressive infantile experience, from which the child tends to exit via a manic defence that establishes itself over time, may find confirmation in those forms of transsexualism that arise in very fragile environmental and family contexts. Suffice to think of the phenomenon of the Brazilian transsexuals who come from the *favelas*. To become a beautiful, admired woman who is also paid because she can give sexual pleasure is obviously more desirable than being a humiliated, deprived child with no future, as happens to those who are obliged to live in dehumanising circumstances.

A very important element in primary transsexualism, as shown by the accounts of treatments of transsexual children, is the pervasive presence of persecutory anxiety that demands the production of defence mechanisms that harm the nascent gender identity. This aspect has been highlighted by many authors, in particular by Oppenheimer (1991), for whom the deficit in perception of one's own masculinity would provoke anxieties of fragmentation, disintegration, and annihilation.

The presence of profound anxiety and a fear of male violence is certainly an important element in the case of the child Renato (Moriggia, note 14), but the same mix emerges in the cases of the young Colin (Coates & Moore, 1997), Antoine (Chiland, 2000), and Jaime (Busch de Ahumada, 2003). In these children, an incapacity to mobilise defences against aggression, especially regarding the male figure, perceived as the bearer of dangerous violence, is clearly evident. It would seem that, in these cases, anxiety is primary and not consequent to the gender identity disorder: that is, to the child's feelings of being alone and different.

To conclude, I would like to recall that gender identity is constructed in the imaginative sphere of the individual, although conditioned by multiple environmental and transgenerational elements. We know that many of our beliefs, while real to us and useful for our existence, can be disclaimed by others. Often, our own identity can be partially imaginary. In fact, the imagination can develop in harmony with psychic (and physical) reality or it can nurture a delusional desire that requires reality (and one's body) to be adapted and transformed, and that will only be realised by, and find relief through, the current surgical techniques.

The therapeutic stories I have recounted clearly show that, in the case of transsexualism, the earlier the therapy begins the more successful the results are likely to be. In childhood, the formation of the identity is still fluid and the transsexual identity has not yet become a psychic reality that sustains the whole personality. This is why it is important to work in childhood: only in this way can we work through the basic anxiety and help the defensive constructions that uphold the transsexual desire to evolve.

While the number of transsexuals is not very high, their clinical cases pose a very complex task for psychoanalysis (Pfäfflin, 2006). We can undoubtedly say that they constitute the prototype of difficult cases.

All the colleagues mentioned in this chapter, to whom I am greatly indebted, prompt us to reflect on the fact that transsexualism obliges us to think analytically in a new way, without being able to rely on what is already known. We are confronting the mysterious foundation of the psychic and bodily self and the complex tangle between what is learnt and what is biologically preordained in the construction of our personality. For this reason, I believe that studies of this sort should not be considered in a marginal light, even if they deal with issues that, for the moment, are not generally part of an analyst's daily clinical work.

CHAPTER TWELVE

Reflections on the origins of sexual perversions

"If I go into a butcher's shop I always think it's surprising that
I wasn't there instead of the animal"

(Francis Bacon in Sylvester, 1998, p. 46)

Perversion can be defined as a technique of mental arousal that
originates in isolation and is nurtured in the imagination.
Sexual pleasure is obtained through specific mental images
linked to the idea of dominating and possessing a person, or, on the
contrary, of being dominated and possessed.

In this chapter, I explore a number of specific environmental
experiences that can meet with a particular disposition in the child
and go on to develop a perversion characterised by self-harm and the
annihilation of vital aggression.

A famous patient

The analysis has essentially established the following:

The physical chastisements administered to the patient's posterior
by her father from the age of four until seven unfortunately became

associated with the patient's premature and now highly developed sexual awareness. This sexuality came to be expressed by the patient from very early on by her rubbing her thighs together to commence an act of masturbation. Masturbation always occurred after she underwent punishment from her father. After a while the beatings were no longer necessary to initiate sexual arousal; it came to be triggered through mere threats and other situations implying violence, such as verbal abuse, threatening movements of the hands, and so on. After a time she could not even look at her father's hands without becoming sexually aroused, or watch him eat without imagining how the food was ejected, and then being thrashed on the buttocks, and so on. These associations extended to the younger brother too, who also masturbated frequently from an early age. Threats to the boy or ill-treatment of him aroused her and she had to masturbate whenever she saw him being punished. In time any situation which reflected violence aroused her, for example, being told to obey. As soon as she was alone she was plagued by obsessional fantasies: for example, she would imagine all kinds of torments. The same happened in her dreams: for example, she often dreamt that she was eating her lunch and simultaneously sitting on the lavatory and that everything was going straight out through her bottom; at the same time she was surrounded by a large crowd of people watching her; on another occasion she was being whipped in front of a great mob of people, and so on.

This clinical account is part of a letter dated 25 September 1905 that Jung sent to Sigmund Freud by way of presenting the case of Sabina Spielrein (Covington & Wharton, 2003, p. 106).

If we recall Freud's paper "'A child is being beaten'" (1919e), we may assert that, in Sabina's case, the masochistic fantasy did not spontaneously arise in her mind but was subsequent to a real traumatic event: the child, in this case, was really beaten.

The relationship between trauma and perversion is not, however, always as linear as the reconstruction of Sabina Spielrein's childhood might lead us to suppose. In her case, it would seem that fear of paternal punishment triggered a state of arousal that was fuelled by perpetual fantasies that Sabina repeated, moreover, in the relationship with those treating her during her hospital stay.

The passionate nature of the future analyst saved her from the fate of retreating into the perversion. In fact, her symptoms disappeared during her therapy with Jung.

Clinical material

Alfredo, a masochistic transvestite, habitually inflicts severe bodily punishment on himself whenever he makes a mistake. Once the error has been identified, he plans a punishment that has to be inflicted as many times as the number on the die thrown. He dreams of having Eichmann, the Nazi criminal, in his pay, who appears to him dressed in white as he is preaching to a group. The confused aspect of the dream regards the denial of the character's criminal nature: dressed in white, Eichmann, attempting to win over converts, would be innocent.

* * *

It is obvious from this dream that the sadistic perverse structure, personified by Eichmann, is considered good and is nurtured by the patient himself (he is on his payroll).

* * *

Bruno, a second sadomasochistic patient in analysis, uses parts of the body to animate sadomasochistic sequences: he tightly binds up his penis and then beats it. The hitting hand represents a sadistic man while the tortured penis stands for an abused young boy. After a brief period of analysis, he dreamt of striking his penis, while the analyst stood by aloof and indifferent.

* * *

In the dream I (analyst) represent the projection of his excited and perverse confusion, but I am also a psychologically absent parental figure, similar to the parents of his past who did not understand nor interfere with his infantile sexualised withdrawal.

At first sight, these two patients seem very similar: both dominated by sadomasochistic excitement and both carried away by the attractions of the perverse. How are they different?

Born with a serious form of hypospadias, Alfredo underwent repeated reconstructive surgery during his first years of life. It is legitimate to think that these interventions, together with the prolonged stays in hospital, were traumatic elements that might have fostered his initiation into masochistic perversion.

However, this is not the case with Bruno, who was born and grew up in a well-off middle-class family and whose childhood was apparently devoid of major traumatic events; but, as his dream testi-fies, he was also an isolated child far from any parental emotional participation.

To return to the actual trauma, it is documented that masochistic fantasies can emerge from early painful somatic intrusions that the child perceives as sadistic aggression.

Glenn (1984) relates the case of three patients who had undergone serious prolonged surgery in infancy and who subsequently devel-oped erotised sadomasochistic fantasies. Similar observations were made by Stoller (1975) of adult patients.

In the Panel "Sadomasochism in children" (1985), a number of observations were reported of premature children who had had to undergo traumatic surgery (Grossman, 1991). The dramatic cases presented document the fact that an extraordinary capacity to respond to trauma with erotised masochistic behaviour develops in early infancy.

The trauma

The consequences of precocious traumatic infantile experiences on the development of pathologies and suffering destined to become mani-fest in adulthood are considered in many ways. The difficulties begin when one tries to establish which experiences should be considered traumatic in the individual case, also because the evaluation can only be made afterwards. How the traumatic experience is worked through depends largely on the response of the adults who are looking after the child. If there is a constant and understanding affective parental presence, the consequences of the trauma will be diminished. For this reason, the relationship between early trauma and the subsequent development of a perversion is somewhat complex.

As well as physical aggression, such as being hit or sadistic acts, the child can be exposed to sexual traumas, such as episodic or repea-ted sexual violence. However, the most frequent cause of an adult's perverse behaviour does not seem to lie with the more serious trau-mas (ill-treatment, violence, or sexual abuse). This type of violent trauma causes considerable damage to the child's personality, but it is found more in borderline cases and personality disorders of a delin-quent type.

The hypothesis I will present in this chapter is that, apart from the cases involving surgery in early infancy that I have mentioned above, it is not traumas of a violent nature that lure a person towards perversion; on the contrary, it is a profound emotional absence that encourages a *sexualised withdrawal*. It might be said that this is the *traumatic* element that prepares the ground for the perverse experience in the adult.

These states of sexualised withdrawal develop early on as defences against experiences of emptiness and are connected to the nature of the primary objects and to their interaction with the patient.

* * *

Corrado, who came to analysis for a serious form of depression and anxiety that led him to frequent stays in psychiatric hospitals, reveals that since he was very small he has been erotically attracted to women's feet. Even now, this is the stimulus for his irresolute sexuality. The infantile image that emerges in analysis shows a child entrusted to a constant turnover of nannies who remembers the countless times he went into his mother's room and saw her varnish her toenails red before some social event. Corrado remembers the excitement this vision gave him. Another infantile memory shows him lying down with his mother, who is engrossed in watching television while he caresses her feet and fantasies a sexual relationship with her; at the same time he squeezes his penis between his thighs and reaches (mental) orgasm.

* * *

Ever since he was tiny, the foot has been the only accessible part of his mother's body; in her indifference, she lets it sexually arouse her child. It is interesting to note that, in this case, the foot fetish developed at an early age, when a lack of affective maternal participation was replaced by eroticised arousal. Even today, Corrado still goes to porn clubs where he watches sex shows through peepholes or lightly touches the body (better bodies) of the women who exhibit themselves to his voyeuristic arousal.

* * *

Dino is another foot fetishist. He is young, very depressed and passive, and his life lacks all meaning. He has constant masochistic relations with women, with whom he fantasies annulling himself, putting himself totally in their hands. Another compulsory masochistic behaviour, an attempt to throw off the anxiety that assails him, is to have sex with a prostitute who has been specifically chosen for her unappealing appearance.

In analysis, Dino is often engulfed by fantasies of submission and annihilation and speaks forcefully of his fetishist fantasy: for him, women's feet are tantamount to possessing a treasure and are part of the neo-created reality that disburses a totalising pleasure. His arousal (linked to something dirty and foetid) relates to anal masturbation, although it is connected to a fantasy of annihilation (under a woman's feet).

* * *

Dino's pathology is the outcome of a particular childhood story in which the affective absence of his parents—bound together by a narcissistic bond—prevented sufficient psychological closeness with their son, condemning him to solitude.

Masochistic fantasies

When they are frankly pathological, family relationships obviously play a part in creating damage.

For a young girl to see her parents in sadomasochistic collusion (the mother apparently consenting to be dominated by the husband who sexually abuses her) reinforces in her mind the idea of a sadistic penis and of a relationship based on disparity; the impression that sexual relations occur without reciprocal pleasure is strengthened. If this is the emotional world the girl lives in, it is easy to imagine what her sexual experience may be as an adult.

* * *

A patient of mine, Elvira, was unable to experience pleasure in her relations with her boyfriend unless she imagined him having sex with another woman. In her fantasy, she was part of the scene although she did not take part. She could not experience pleasure at first hand, only being able to reach it through a voyeuristic fantasy. This allowed her to feel a state of arousal in which sexual desire was not lived as guilty, since the pleasure belonged to someone else.

Another variant on masochistic pleasure was to imagine herself abused by a violent man. It was clear that Elvira was completely immersed in the sadomasochistic relationship that had characterised her parents' relationship and that she had identified with her mother, who was probably frigid but who appeared submissive in the face of her husband's domination. Elvira's partner was unconsciously felt to be the intrusive, psychologically and physically violent father.

This parental couple, at least as far as it was experienced by the patient, had been the premise for the emergence of a sadomasochistic fantasy in which the state of submission was sexualised.

* * *

In many cases of frigidity and of masochistic fantasies that lead to pleasure, it is discovered that the lack of a good relationship between the parental couple prevents the development of infantile sexual imagination.

These patients are unable to reach sexual enjoyment because they cannot explore and project their desires for pleasure. The masochistic fantasy relates back to the emotional trauma that marked this delicate and sensitive sphere of sexuality. I believe that this type of infantile psychic trauma plays an important role in creating areas of suffering in the adult's amorous life and is at the basis of various forms of female sexual masochism. Preventing the development of the capacity for sexual enjoyment, the trauma channels it towards masochistic pleasure: whoever suffered passively can now derive active pleasure.

In some women, frigidity subsequent to infantile sexual abuse can be circumvented by marshalling fantasies of self-annihilation. In these cases, we are not dealing with true perversion, but with manoeuvres directed at attaining orgasm during normal sexual relations.

Even in cases where abuse has led to sexualised behaviour, this is not to be confused with perversion.

A child sexually abused by an adult suffers a catastrophic attack on his trust in the world that threatens his capacity to believe in the good dependence of human objects. Sexual abuse is the most serious form of adult betrayal of a child (Parens, 1997) and is destined to produce a series of inhibitions in the personality of whoever suffers it.

Sexual trauma and seduction by adults induce the child to face the processes of growth by dissociating the experience of the abuse

(Davies, 1996), which may float to consciousness later on in life or during therapy.

The emotional disorder

As said above, for the perversion to form, seductive or authoritarian pressure from an adult (usually the mother) on the mind of the child is often necessary, as, in that way, his perception of independence and separateness is attacked.

This type of traumatic interference has been explained in various ways. Childhood micro-traumas, which Khan (1979) refers to with his concept of cumulative trauma, can contribute to creating various character areas of a narcissistic or self-erotic type that, according to the author, become specific elements in the development of perversion in adulthood.

Other authors believe that perversions depend on an infantile "withdrawal" subsequent to the parents' emotional distancing; the case described by Joseph (1982) in her paper "Addiction to near death" falls within this line of interpretation.

The trauma–perversion sequence can even be overturned and lead us to suppose that in children secretly devoted to sadomasochistic withdrawal, the traumatic experiences can give rise to sexual pleasure. In these cases, the trauma, instead of being experienced as a source of anxiety, reawakens sadistic pleasure and stirs up the masochistic fantasy.

Bruno, the patient I have already discussed above, related that once, as a child, he was approached and touched up by an elderly paedophile, from whom he ran away, frightened. Despite this, that evening he made up an excited fantasy in which he sucked the old man's dirty penis.

The trauma had inserted itself into a perverse readiness that was already present, opening up the path towards the excited masochistic fantasy.

Edoardo, instead, is a masochistic patient in which no trace of trauma exists. He came to me because he had read my book on sado-masochism (De Masi, 2003[1999]) and had been struck on recognising many aspects of himself in it.

*   *   *

Edoardo has always lived in a family that can be called normal, and had an intense relationship with his mother while his father was always experienced as a distant figure. He says that his first memory involving perversion dates back to his earliest years, when, very small, he was playing with robots. Once, one of these had been tied up to stop it escaping and he had found this constricted state arousing. He felt the same sensation on watching cartoons in which two heroine sisters were captured, tied up, and threatened by bandits. During the years of elementary school, he got into the habit of tying himself up and found that it was more exciting if he could wear female clothes or tights that he used to take from his mother. When he dressed up like this he used to stand in front of the mirror and the sight of his body in women's clothes, looking as though it really was a woman tied up and trying to free herself from her bonds, gave him enormous pleasure. Even today, Edoardo loses himself in fantasies of slavery and is still not clear if what excites him the most is to submit or to be the dominator.

*   *   *

The family context he grew up in was characterised by his parents' silent presence. I have already mentioned his father: a man regularly away at work, of few words, and with an elementary, although not bad, psychology. His mother was more present, but not very capable of structuring a growing young boy; she wanted a son who studied, and he did that, but she never seemed worried during his adolescence about the absence of friends or his lack of interest in people of his own age. Edoardo is certain that his mother "knows" about his customary practices, and remembers a time when he was surprised by his mother while he was tied up, but she never said a word about it.

The trauma sexualised

At times, the emotional trauma that verges towards perversion does not derive from the parents' emotional distance, as in the case described above, but, instead, from their intrusive pathogenic presence.

At this point I would like to report in greater detail the analytic material of a patient to show the link between psychic trauma and the perverse construction.

In this case, the outcome of the perversion did not depend only on the presence of a pathological parent, but also on the fact that the emotional trauma was sexualised. In other words, a psychopathological construction developed alongside the emotional trauma in which the very significance of the violence suffered was lost.

*   *   *

Even if Carlo, married and with two children, was on drugs at the beginning of the analysis, his real addiction was to masochistic fantasies. He had always been very ill ever since he was small, and had grown up without a father (who had died when he was very young) in an excessively intimate but, at the same time, frustrating relationship with his mother. She used to keep him with her in bed at night when she was alone, ready to move him out as soon as she had a lover. The absence of a paternal figure was crucial and led the patient to despair that a filial relationship with the analyst could constitute an experience of emotional growth.

The dominant pathological structure was characterised by the fact that, instead of separating from his mother, Carlo became a totally passive prisoner as far as she was concerned. Precisely due to this pleasure for transforming activity into passivity, he confessed he was incapable of educating his own children, who subjected him to all sorts of abuse. He lived in a state of constant perverse withdrawal in which he could annihilate affects, emotions, and conflicts by virtue of masturbatory pleasure reached in fantasy. The patient seemed to repeat the same behaviour over and over: incapable of entering into conflict with his relational object, he transformed his anger into an action against himself, treating his infantile self as a slave. In fact, continual fantasies of being reduced to slavery and subjugated to some powerful body (usually a woman) coloured his imagination: these fantasies were accompanied by masturbation or anal penetration with the use of a variety of objects. A part of his life free from sadomasochistic fantasies, and of which he could be proud, was his ability to write and his love for literature.

Often, after a good session, his compulsive sexuality increased. The figure of the analyst was very weak, destined to dwindle rapidly during the separations. At these moments he was taken over not only by masturbatory fantasies, but also, once again, by his improper use of drugs that held him in a state of mental euphoria. Both the sexualised fantasies and the drugs had the objective of emptying his mind and concealing the conflicts and bitter truths of the analytic relationship.

Expressions of appreciation for the benefits obtained in analysis (for example, greater firmness with regard to his children) alternated with flight and masturbatory withdrawal, with a consequential belittlement of the analytic work.

It became increasingly clear that his flight into the fantasy of being a slave allowed him to obliterate his emotions and his real life of relationships. In this fantasy, he was no longer himself; he became a third person; he no longer had any will or emotions; he entered another world. This wiping out of his identity gave him real pleasure; it was a truly erotic experience. Consequently, by morning he felt so empty that he had to masturbate in order to arouse himself and feel a bit more active. To fuel his masochistic fantasies he frequently spent hours glued to the television during the day; he identified with figures of slaves or tried to contact people on the Internet who acted the role of master. When the withdrawal into his perverse fantasy prevailed, the analyst was placed in the position of passive spectator, a voyeur of his arousal. Over time, and with progress made in the analysis, these fantasies began to cease being a source of pleasure; the patient began to avoid them, and when they returned he was filled with anxiety. This was real progress that led to a transformation in Carlo's internal world; he became capable of distinguishing what was pleasurable and exciting from what was useful and good for growth. The perverse fantasy began to be contained by his healthy part.

Another important change occurred towards the fourth year of analysis in a series of sessions in which his pathological relationship with his mother became increasingly clear to him.

In one of these sessions, Carlo began to talk about a fantasy that he had tried to act out with his wife: she was the Queen of Saba and he prostrated himself at her feet. He had remembered that, when small, after seeing the film *Helen of Troy* with his mother, he had had a similar fantasy. While his mother had become the beautiful Greek woman, he had identified with her slave.

Suddenly, he began to lash out at women, all whores, who seduced only despicable men. He then got extremely angry with his mother, insulting her and calling her a "whore". He screamed that she had castrated him, that she had treated him like a girl, taking him to bed with her and making him attend all her parties with her girlfriends.

*   *   *

This series of sessions was important because the patient could begin to confront his hatred for his mother and his custom of prostrating himself before her. Until this moment, he had been unable to experience his negative feelings towards her, erased by the fantasy of submission. He began to realise that while he was ready, in fantasy, to prostrate himself in front of his mother-queen, in reality he hated her. He recognised that she had seduced him, and had never truly loved him. She had never fully valued him and had always chosen other men with whom he, a child, could never hope to compete. She had hysterically considered him a small appendage of herself, a small penis of hers, and not a person. He understood, then, why he slipped so frequently into masochistic fantasies. If it was impossible to have an equal relationship with his mother, and if he should always be in a position of inferiority, then it was best if he submitted to it and completely annihilated himself and enjoyed his own annihilation.

For a long time, the patient incessantly expressed hatred for women, all considered whores; his campaign against them was relentless because he wanted to get the analyst on his side; he wanted the analyst to think like him.

To hate his mother and all the female gender could represent an initial step towards reaching a certain degree of separation from the female figure, but, above all, it was a defence against his feeling of guilt. If all women were whores, then the blame for his perversion was his mother's, not his. If he had admitted that there were perhaps some good relations with a female figure, then he could have been to blame for his failure. He had never been capable of psychically separating from the pathological relationship with his mother and from his relationship of aroused submission, and perhaps had never wanted to; this was what he was guilty of.

If Carlo had been traumatised by a hysterical mother, it was also true that part of his perversion lay precisely in continuing to destroy every good aspect not only in his object, but in all the objects and in himself. He admired women's cruelty and coldness and confused their arrogance with strength. For a long time, Carlo held to his pessimistic cynical view of life: he needed to demonstrate that the world was all bad and that his perversion was justified.

However, during the analytic process, this patient gradually succeeded in freeing himself from the perverse arousal and from the pathological and annihilating relationship with women and stopped projecting everything negative on to the female figure. He then recognised that no one had helped or protected him during his development. The relationship with the analyst became increasingly important because it helped to develop a true personal identity.

The links between trauma and perversion are complex and articulated, and require extremely attentive scrutiny. A connection between them can be grasped *a posteriori* when, on formulating reconstructive hypotheses about the patient's past and identifying with him, one can truly comprehend his story and his journey.

A series of reflections can be proffered from the examination of the clinical cases presented.

As I have attempted to show, there is no connection between violent trauma and perversion. Even if it is documented that some children who have had to bear traumatic suffering during the first years of life (especially surgery) have erotised the pain, perversion, instead, would seem to be facilitated by a complex interweaving of intrafamily emotional disorders.

I believe we can agree on the fact that a certain family constellation is frequently encountered, but the subjective readiness of some children to develop the psychopathological structures that will lead to perversion still remains a mystery.

As I have said, a lack of understanding on the part of the family environment can be pathogenic, but, in some cases, the facilitating and active action of a disordered parent is decisive. This was the case for Carlo, whose adhesion to, and identification with, a pathological maternal figure played an important role. It is also clear, in his case, how the sexualisation of the trauma had, for a long time, obliterated the emotional awareness of the trauma itself and, with it, also the perception of pain and anger.

In short, it seems to me that the perversion is facilitated by the absence of any support for growth on the part of adults, along with their eventual pathological intrusion, rather than by the violent infantile trauma responsible for other serious pathologies.

In any case, the lack of parental participation is answered in the child by flight towards arousal, which serves to replace the relational void. This fosters the start of pathological identifications and structures destined to impede development, as well as a distancing from reality and from relational love.

CHAPTER THIRTEEN

The perverse fascination of the destructive organisation*

"The war of absolute enmity knows no bracketing. The consistent fulfillment of absolute enmity provides its own meaning and justification"

(Schmitt, 2007[1963], p. 36)

I n this chapter, I explore the difference between aggressive violence and destructiveness. Aggression can be thought of as a force that carries out a defensive function and that dies away once its aim has been achieved. Destructiveness, directed at attacking the good objects and at triumphing over human relationships, aims purely at pleasure in and of itself and tends to repeat itself in a drugged way.

Although psychoanalytic thought has long concerned itself with aggression, it has never achieved a unified conception of this subject, but has instead formulated a variety of contrasting theories. Two basic

---

* This paper was read at the Second International Psychoanalytic Conference held in Belfast, May 2010. Translated by Philip Slotkin, MA, Cantab. MITI.

positions can be distinguished. According to the first, aggression (with its corollaries of hate and destructiveness) forms part of the human instinctual endowment, while the second holds that it is a consequence of frustration and trauma.

The champions of the first position include Sigmund Freud and Melanie Klein. Freud saw aggression as an innate component of libido—that is, of the force that presses for the achievement of pleasure and the conquest of objects. Klein (1932), on the other hand, held that the conflict between love and hate (the latter being an expression of the destructive instinct) was the engine of development and the foundation of mental functioning.

The second group of psychoanalysts, who regard aggression as a response to a traumatic experience (that is, deprivation of basic needs or exposure to violence), includes Anna Freud, Fairbairn, Winnicott, Kohut, and, recently, Fonagy.

In this chapter, I attempt to distinguish aggression, which can assume the form of hate and violence, from destructiveness. In so doing, I shall follow Glasser (1998) in distinguishing between self-preservative and sadomasochistic or malignant violence. The former is a type of reactive aggression, directed against a real or imaginary threat; the latter, instead, is a planned act of violence with no regard for affects that occurs in psychopathic personalities. Whereas aggression can be regarded in certain contexts as a defence useful for survival, destructiveness is directed against the very roots of life. In the sphere of mental phenomena, destructiveness underlies severe psychopathologies, such as perversion, anorexic and borderline syndromes, drug addiction, and psychoses. In the social and political field, destructiveness was responsible for the greatest tragedies of the past century, such as Nazism and the derivatives of ideological communism.

Hate

Hate, a feeling that is inevitably present in human beings, is charged with the wish to harm one's adversary. Hating means wanting to cause the object that harms us to suffer and wanting to destroy that object. The difference between reactive and destructive aggression lies not in the intensity of the hate, which might be extreme in both cases, but in the quality and character of the attacked object. Hate is defensive when turned against a bad object, but destructive if the aim is to destroy a good object.

The definition of a good object is, of course, problematic: is a good object one that is useful and gives pleasure, or is it one that gives rise to unpleasure and sometimes pain?

According to Freud (1915c), hate comes before love:

> The ego hates, abhors and pursues with intent to destroy all objects which are a source of unpleasurable feeling for it, without taking into account whether they mean a frustration of sexual satisfaction or of the satisfaction of self-preservative needs. Indeed, it may be asserted that the true prototypes of the relation of hate are derived not from sexual life, but from the ego's struggle to preserve and maintain itself. (p. 138)

A little later, he writes, "Hate, as a relation to objects, is older than love. It derives from the narcissistic ego's primordial repudiation of the external world with its outpouring of stimuli" (p. 139).

From this point of view, hate will be aroused by any stimulus that disturbs the primitive ego's maintenance of pleasure. The narcissistic ego makes no distinction between the inevitable frustration that is necessary for growth and an intentional, malevolent attack; in the narcissistic position, any object that interferes with personal well-being is bad.

People who act violently are often found to be linked to their victims in a sadomasochistic circuit. Hate, which stems from a narcissistic wound or an injustice sustained, is always an unpleasant feeling that is hard to tolerate. Recrimination and ill will excite violence to an uncontainable pitch. By killing, the murderer severs the negative bond between him and his object. Violence is resorted to for internal reasons, to expel an intolerable state of mind, and relief is obtained by ridding oneself not so much of one's enemy as of an intolerable mental state.

Hate is sometimes bound up with anxiety aroused when a person feels humiliated, ignored, or threatened (whether in objective or subjective reality).

Emotional indifference

Destructiveness differs from aggression in that it expresses indifference and lack of hostility towards a specific object; it is an anti-relational operation that takes place in silence, is planned, and develops in a special mental state in which feelings and emotions are abolished. It is possible to be destructive without hating, for hate is unpleasurable and entails conflict, whereas destructive sadism is pleasurable.

It is not always easy to distinguish between these two concepts in the psychoanalytic literature, even in the work of Freud himself, and they are sometimes found to overlap.

In Carol Reed's fine film *The Third Man*, Orson Welles plays the character of Harry Lime, an unscrupulous racketeer wanted by the police in immediate post-war Vienna, then under Russian and American occupation. His old friend Holly Martins (Joseph Cotten), unaware of Harry's activities, arrives in Vienna to look him up just a few days after he has seemingly been killed in a road accident.

Holly is unconvinced by the official version of events and, after many vicissitudes, finds out from certain clues that Harry is alive, but does not know that his friend pretended to be dead so that he could operate undisturbed, without fear of detection by the police who had been hunting for him.

Concerned that his cover has been blown by Holly, Harry decides to meet him in secret; he wants to learn how much his friend knows. He intends to eliminate him before he can talk to the police.

They meet at the Prater amusement park in Vienna, where, in order not to be overheard, the two men take a ride on the giant Ferris wheel. When the pod reaches its highest point, Harry, who has been contemplating getting rid of his friend by thrusting him out and causing him to plunge to the ground, says to him, "Take a look down below: if one of those dots you see down there were to disappear, would you feel sorry? If I were to offer you £2000 for every dot that disappeared, would you tell me to keep my money? Or would you count how many dots were left?"

This memorable scene describes one of the possible versions of the process of dehumanisation. The mental condition concerned could be defined in terms of Harry Lime's statement that men are little dots that can be eliminated. With the seduction of power and contempt for the shared values of solidarity, Lime attempts to corrupt Martins; in other words, he tries to use the same arguments that seduced his own mind as propaganda. His words express a cynical, perverse attitude in which empathy with the fate of others is totally lacking. Perversion coincides neither with aggression nor with hate, but is the absence of love—that is, indifference. Its nucleus is pleasurable destructiveness, which thrives in indifference and the absence of passion.

Dehumanisation

Nowadays, achievement of the mental state of emotional indifference, which underlies the process of dehumanisation, is facilitated by the use of technology, which enables a person to kill without the perception of killing.

> They are so remote from their so-called enemies, and they have to aim from such a distance, that they are no longer really *aiming*; they no longer have any perception of their victims, they have no knowledge of them, and cannot even imagine them. Not before, not while it is happening, and not afterwards. Can such things be called *soldiers*? And how could such soldiers hate people they have never met and (considering that they will have been eliminated) never will meet? And these soldiers, who no longer engage in hand-to-hand combat, who no longer share a battlefield with the enemy, but are at best manipulating instruments in some ill-defined place from which not a single enemy soldier is within sight – why would these soldiers need hate? Is it not, would it not be, an utterly superfluous feeling? One that is absolutely outdated? (Anders, 1985, translated for this edition)

This long extract is taken from an essay whose title translates as "The outdatedness of hating", by an author who always spoke out against war and the destructiveness of man, and who drew particular attention to the danger of dehumanisation that is characteristic of our age.

Sharing of emotions

It was Ferenczi, in "The unwelcome child and his death-instinct" (1929), who had the insight that linked the death wish to infantile emotional trauma: in this contribution, he postulates that the lack of vitality and the wish to disappear into the void that characterise certain lives have their origin in the child's conscious or unconscious perception of maternal rejection. In view of the important role of the earliest infantile experiences in strengthening or weakening the vital aspects of the personality, it will readily be understood that a child exposed at an early stage to psychologically unfavourable events might ultimately tend to destroy the life drive within him. Similarly, where the conditions of dependence impose intolerable suffering on an individual, a wish for self-annihilation might be the response to prolonged exposure to trauma.

Certain findings of neuroscientific research confirm long-established insights by psychoanalysts, who are in continuous touch with the human mind. The neurosciences are, at present, particularly concerned with the problem of how human minds perceive each other and how feelings are transmitted from individual to individual. After all, a human being's capacity to communicate his emotions allows his interlocutor to share in and feel something of the relevant experience for himself without, thereby, forfeiting his separateness. That is the only way an individual can respond empathically to a fellow human being and help him.

Rizzolatti and colleagues (2001) discovered the existence of *mirror neurons*, a group of nerve cells that are activated when we see someone perform an action involving movement. In other words, certain cell groups begin to resonate and activate the same muscles in the observer as those used by the person who is at that time performing a purposive action. This kind of activation is not equivalent to the initiation of an *imitative process*, but instead tends to establish sensorimotor procedures that are unconsciously learnt in the early phases of life; their unconscious repetition facilitates access to a motor alphabet that permits a better understanding of the intention of the person performing the relevant action.

The same mechanism, based on a preparedness to internalise and reproduce what is perceived of the other, may underlie the ways in which the individual learns to apprehend not only the meaning of actions, but also other people's sensations or emotions.

The place in the mind that enables us to understand others emotionally comes into being because we have been understood in turn and have fully internalised the experience of emotional contact with the other. In order to be born and to develop as individuals, we must have been received emotionally in the mind of an adult (primordially, that of the mother).

The quality of the parental response can either help a child to acquire a realistic self-perception that will enable him to relate to the world or stimulate him to negate truth and to develop an altered, grandiose, narcissistic personality. The mother might see her child as exceptional and make him believe he is special, destined to become master of the world. Such an attitude reinforces grandiosity and legitimises the assumption of being privileged and consequent arrogance. The adult subject will then remain in the paranoid–schizoid mental position and regard anyone who threatens his supposed superiority as an enemy.

Omnipotence and destructiveness

The prolific Swiss psychoanalyst Alice Miller (1983) wondered why the children of violent, abusive parents tended in turn to ill-treat others. An unloved or unwanted child is potentially destined to become a violent adult who will take revenge on others for the traumas he has sustained or who will beat his own children, and, thus, is likely to generate further oppressors or criminals-to-be. In Miller's view, a child's aggression is positive, necessary for survival, and derived from the life instinct; it is events subsequent to birth that result in negative psychic development. Since a traumatic environment calls for the suppression of feelings and idealisation of the aggressors, a child in this situation will grow up without developing an awareness of what was done to him. His split-off feelings of anger, impotence, and despair will continue to find expression in destructive acts against others (criminality) or himself (drug addiction, alcoholism, prostitution, mental disorders, or suicide). In her passionate defence of the ill-treated child, the Swiss analyst also examines the case of Adolf Hitler, who, as a child, was constantly beaten by his father. Miller claims that the German dictator's traumatic infancy partly explains the destructive nature of his political leadership.

In my opinion, Alice Miller does not sufficiently emphasise that, although in conflict with his father, Hitler enjoyed the boundless admiration of his mother and, later, of his sister, and that this maternal exaltation might have fuelled his conviction of being a superman. In other words, I take the view that the relationship between trauma and the process of dehumanisation is not always so straightforward. It is not only trauma that favours human destructiveness; seduction by grandiose figures who cause confusion between good and evil could be even more telling. In such cases, a part of the personality justifies the destructive behaviour in the name of a moral imperative. The individual is then subordinated to a value system that stems from a perversion of conscience. That is the psychological condition of Harry Lime, the protagonist of *The Third Man*, discussed earlier.

The psychotic part of the personality

Rosenfeld (1971) and Meltzer (1973) advance the hypothesis that a mental structure that wins over the healthy parts of the personality with seductive propaganda, then colonising it and impelling it towards destructiveness, is responsible for the more serious psychic pathologies.

This pathological structure, which causes the most complex forms of mental suffering, has been variously referred to by the terms *destructive narcissism* or the *psychotic part of the personality*. The most insidious aspect of this mental state is the lack of any clear awareness of its pathological aims, which can even be regarded as inevitable and aspirational. The impelling move towards the pathological behaviour proceeds in secrecy and silence; indeed, a deadly force presenting idealised, exciting, and positive traits dominates the personalities of these patients. When working with them, it is important to distinguish the vital aggression from the aggression connected to the narcissistic organisation, which is directed against the emotive self and the good objects. In other words, from the destructiveness deriving from the pathological organisation and tantamount to a silent, hidden force, relentless and deadly, as I will show in the case history of Alfredo, below.

In order to keep excitation alive, the perverse action must constantly increase the dose of "badness". A work of literature in which this is demonstrated is Sade's "The one hundred and twenty days of Sodom" (1991). Just when the libertines have their victims completely at their mercy and can do anything they like with them, including killing them, they realise that they are habituated to excitation; they then recognise that, however much they raise the pitch of violence, they will never be satisfied. The real crime, rather than a sequence of wretched misdeeds, would be to put out the sun in order to destroy the universe.

Analytical clinical work

Fifteen-year-old Alfredo was sent for therapy by his parents when they learnt from one of his schoolmates that he intended to commit suicide. A highly intelligent youngster who did not look anything like a normal adolescent, he dressed in black like an old man (he wore a double-breasted jacket and black shoes) and behaved accordingly. As was discovered during the course of the therapy, his parents had always remained emotionally remote from him. His upbringing with them had been cold, dutiful, and, in many respects, crushing. His only significant relationship had been with his grandfather, who had cared for him but had treated him like an adult, thus stimulating the logical and mathematical aspects of his intelligence.

Alfredo had always been an isolated child who did not like to play with others of his own age. Even now he had no friends. He excelled academically and had a privileged relationship only with his teachers, who were often astonished by his intellectual performance. When he grew up he wanted to be a doctor, not because he wished to help the suffering, but because he aspired to the role of anatomist/pathologist so that he could dissect corpses.

During his first few sessions, Alfredo mentioned several times that he spent many hours of his day designing a bunker in which he wished to live. In this refuge he would be able to create all the reality he wanted; this reality could be magnificent (he was a scientist or a famous mathematician), but also bloody and grim. He fantasised that in his bunker he was a great surgeon who could disfigure or cut into his patients or tear them to pieces. The withdrawal into fantasy had recently become so invasive that he was afraid of being utterly colonised by it. He confessed that, in class, he allowed himself to be carried away by these fantasies to such an extent that he would lose touch with his fellow pupils and his teachers.

Alfredo's mind had now been well and truly taken over by the pleasure of violence and the thrill of blood. He announced that he had begun to eat raw meat, and in his sessions he showed the analyst the cuts he had inflicted on his body; he also described certain fantasies which came to him in his bunker-cum-mortuary and which had the power to excite him. In one of them, he was working as an anatomist/ pathologist in a disused, dilapidated hospital with blood everywhere. A voice called him by a German name; the woman on whom he was operating was not at all dead, even though she was nailed to the operating table. He had given her a very fine nose, but, just when his work was finished, he was seized by an irresistible impulse. While being complimented by the nurse, he decided to demolish the patient's entire face because it seemed to him to be flabby. His scalpel savagely disfigured the woman's face, leaving it bathed in blood. In the second part of the fantasy, a girl led him into a dark corridor. She was accompanied by a French poodle. Alfredo ordered her to kill it. The girl did not want to sacrifice her pet, stroked it and wept. He insisted. The girl began to wring the puppy's neck; although in tears, she broke its neck. The sound of the bones breaking could be heard. At the moment when the girl killed the dog, Alfredo felt pleasure.

* * *

Since his earliest infancy Alfredo had succeeded in fleeing from emotional reality and taking refuge in pathological withdrawal (a megalomaniac state of being flushed with power). In this psychic retreat, pathological identifications took place with grandiose, destructive characters, such as the hangman, the dictator, the great surgeon, and the anatomist/pathologist. In deploying all his omnipotence, Alfredo distorted reality.

The serial killer

It was astonishing to observe the sequence of events that could have led this young man to become a serial killer. In one session, Alfredo produced an extremely insightful description of the relationship between destructiveness and destructive pleasure: "Maybe I like this stuff because it makes me powerful . . . I imagine myself as a powerful person like a hangman . . . a doctor . . . a dictator; I spend the whole day in my imaginary bunker. I'm always a dictator with my army or a mad surgeon . . . what makes me happiest is to be a hangman, as I hold people's lives in my hands; having someone's life in my hands, I like that . . . it amuses me until I decide to kill them. When I imagine myself as a dictator, I am living in a huge bunker; there aren't many other people—apart from myself, there are just the guards and my family . . . then I imagine all the stylish furnishings . . . I spend hours just imagining."

Alfredo was obviously getting more and more fascinated by the possibility of becoming a diabolical being, and this frightened even him. Dehumanisation, the fascination of the negative, the pleasure in blood and death, and the ecstasy of destruction—all these elements were taking him over and beginning to form part of a new and dangerous personality. The puppy that was killed was not only the good infantile part that succumbed to the diabolical part that took pleasure in destruction, but also his infantile aggressive vitality, which had been extinguished. In his relational life, for example with his schoolmates, Alfredo could not tolerate any conflict. In any contest or situation of rivalry or jealousy, he would give way, but would then spend hours in fantasies about torturing his enemy, tearing him to pieces or dissecting him.

This behaviour greatly facilitates understanding of the difference between aggression and destructiveness: Alfredo was not at all *aggressive*; he was unable to assert himself with his schoolmates, to make demands on them, or to defend himself if he was attacked by them. On the contrary, he was constantly engaged in imagining acts of *destructive cruelty* that fuelled and exalted his omnipotent self.

The risk in his case was that he himself might fall victim to his mad part, from which the fascination with murder and the pleasure of destructiveness stemmed, so that he was liable to attack and harm himself.

Criminality and perversion

There is voluminous psychoanalytic literature on criminality and perversion, on the connections between them and on their distinguishing features. Freud postulates that the sexual pleasure obtained by a pervert can mitigate aggression. According to another interpretation, however, the fact that pleasure is achieved through violence makes that violence more redoubtable and dangerous.

I shall now describe a perversion which gradually turned into actual criminal behaviour, and that may be regarded as evidence in favour of the second hypothesis. The description is taken from the notes of the social worker in charge of Jürgen Bartsch, whose case is described in Alice Miller's *For Your Own Good* (1983).

After a number of failed attempts, Jürgen Bartsch finally succeeded in killing four youths aged between sixteen and twenty. Even if each crime varied in detail, the basic procedure was always the same: having lured the youth into an old air-raid shelter, Jürgen would beat him, terrorise him into a totally submissive state, tie him up, manipulate his genitals, and finally strangle him or beat him to death.

Although Jürgen himself and the doctors who surgically castrated him believed the contrary, sexuality seems to have had little to do with the motivation of his criminal acts. Jürgen confessed that, from the age of thirteen or fourteen, his mind had been increasingly disturbed, so that he was ultimately powerless to influence the events that were to overwhelm him. For a long time he prayed, hoping that this at least might be of some help. He reported that he was particularly aroused by the dazed eyes of his victims: paralysed with terror, these young men became so small and submissive that they were unable to protest or defend themselves in any way. The victims' helplessness inflamed the aggressor's sadism even more. (Miller, 1983, pp. 198–239)

According to the detailed description given to the court, the acme of excitation was attained not during masturbation, but only when the victim's body was cut. This meticulous operation gave rise to a kind of permanent mental orgasm. There is not enough information to reconstruct the progressive and inexorable seizure of power by the sadistic, murderous part over the rest of Jürgen's personality. Since feelings of friendship and brotherhood for his young companions persisted in other parts of his person, he must surely have struggled to rein in and neutralise the perverse part of himself. Ultimately, however, just as his victims appeared submissive and incapable of defence, so the good part of his personality became totally helpless and colluded with the murderous part.

This case history presented by Miller, despite the summary nature of the autobiographical account, confirms that—in some cases, at least—the achievement of lustful mental pleasure underlies the criminal impulse.

I do not know why the acting out of cruelty and the infliction of suffering give rise to orgasmic mental excitation. I can only record the fact that the link with sexual ecstasy makes cruelty increasingly devastating and dangerous. This type of pleasure seems totally detached from the sexual act and the associated gratification (libido), and is, therefore, inconsistent with the Freudian paradigm. Destructiveness triumphs through the criminal act because such an act can trigger this type of pleasure.

The pleasure of destructive sexuality

"I maintain that sexuality is an immensely wide field that has never been fully explored." These are the words not of an academic, but of Gianfranco Stevanin, a serial killer who committed his crimes in a small village near Verona. Stevanin killed a number of prostitutes, whom he lured to his farm, where he dismembered their bodies and buried them. When he described the committing of his murders to the court assessor, the memory could apparently arise only when he was in a trance-like state.

Recalling his crimes as if they had been carried out in a state of altered consciousness seemed to be not only a convenient defence against the criminal charges. Stevanin had, in fact, probably been gradually colonised by a particular type of criminal sexuality and had then committed terrible acts without any awareness of what he was doing. This murderer is mentioned here in order to show that perverse fantasy can not only drive a person to commit criminal acts, but also give rise to a quasi-hypnoid state of dissociated consciousness. Having been committed, Stevanin's criminal acts were dissociated from the memory of them, and, as it were, buried with the bodies of the hapless murdered women. Indeed, he might well have obtained a particular kind of pleasure from dissecting his victims' corpses. This, of course, is reminiscent of young Alfredo's fantasies and of Jürgen Bartsch.

"You can do anything you like!"

What is the origin of the pleasure of doing evil—of perverse criminal pleasure? Homicidal destructiveness is attributable not to hate (neither Stevanin nor Bartsch hated their victims), but to its allowing the maximum possible degree of licence and transgressive omnipotence: "You can do anything you like; you can even kill!" Hence, the possible escalation of perversion into a criminal act is due to factors inherent in the nature and dynamics of perverse pleasure and not to hatred of the object. A perverse individual commits crime in the world of fantasy and fiction, whereas a criminal pervert does so in actual reality. For this reason, the connection between cruelty and mental ecstasy is especially dangerous.

According to the British psychoanalyst Arthur Hyatt Williams (1998), who undertook the therapy of criminals, murder is often committed in reality when it has already been perpetrated many times before in waking fantasies or nightmares, and sometimes in unconscious fantasies that have never attained consciousness. This is also partly true of Sade, who, while incarcerated in prison and in an asylum for the criminally insane owing to his sexual excesses and persecution of the authorities, was able to express his unceasing perverse fantasies in concrete form by describing them in his novels. In this way, he could contain the horror in the disturbing fascination of his literary *oeuvre*, without acting it out as he had begun to do and would surely have continued to do had he remained at liberty.

Discussing the problem of masochism and sadism in the context of the death drive, Freud (1924c) points out that masochism is incomprehensible if it is accepted that the pleasure principle—the custodian not only of mental life but of life in general—dominates the mental processes. The pleasure principle is not only the custodian of psychic life, but also of life in general. Masochism would be a great danger, whereas sadism would not. Freud also accepts the existence of a primary masochism, seen as deriving from the holding back of the death drive by the libido, and postulates that destructiveness directed against oneself or others is simply a consequence of the defusion of the libidinal and destructive drives. When the latter are no longer bound and moderated by the former, less and less restraint is placed on their expression.

Rosenfeld (1987) rightly points out that, when fusion occurs, it is a successful attempt by the destructive part to colonise the rest of the personality. In this case, the violence of the destructive impulse is not tempered, but greatly potentiated. A weakness of Freud's theory lies precisely in the difficulty of postulating a meeting or fusion of two antagonistic drives that are destined to cancel each other out.

A more useful model for understanding this fascination invokes the split between the healthy and perverse parts of the personality. However, the two parts are not in static equilibrium, because the perverse part of the personality will eventually colonise the healthy part. This process is clearly visible in the case history of Alfredo, who is taken over by the destructive propaganda to such an extent that it drives him to use his own body as an object on which to enact his murderous impulses. The infantile part, represented by the girl with the puppy, submits masochistically and fails to oppose the pleasure of cruelty and the spilling of blood.

In my view, the psychoanalytic arguments outlined above help not only to identify a comprehensible link between the problem of evil and that of pleasure, but also to explain the degree and quality of the "evil" at work. I have postulated the existence of various sequences or levels seeking to distinguish themselves from each other: there is a psychically "comprehensible" evil and an evil that is utterly remote from any possibility of comprehension.

As Brenman (2006) notes, it gives rise to a specific form of narrow-mindedness without which evil cannot be kept up continuously. His contention is that in order to maintain the practice of cruelty, a singular narrow-mindedness of purpose is put into operation. The consequence of this process produces a cruelty that is "inhuman".

I contend that, unlike hate, destructiveness leads to a form of mental orgasm that allows the subject to act outside the realm of awareness and responsibility. What is involved is a pleasurable destructiveness, which thrives in indifference and the absence of passion: "Rape has nothing to do with impotence. Absolute domination of another body becomes a drug. You rape, torture, and murder for the sense of being the master of other people's fate," said Angelo Izzo, who killed two women after imprisoning them and torturing them and who repeated the same crime after an interval of thirty years, murdering a mother and daughter whom he had befriended while on day release from a semi-custodial sentence.

In this chapter, I have attempted to describe how pleasure is reached in a perverse mental state, in which it is evident that destructiveness encourages mental excitation that makes evil seem pleasurable and irresistible. Hence, Sacher-Masoch's (1947) specific emphasis on the "over-sensitive" and "over-sensual" character of perverse pleasure. Ecstatic and sensual pleasure is bound up with evil, by which it is fuelled.

CHAPTER FOURTEEN

Pathological dependences on the Internet

"Why should one tell the truth if it's to one's advantage to tell a lie?"

(Wittgenstein, a note written at the
age of nine, in Sparti, 2000, p. 23)

P athological dependences on the Internet have reached worrying
levels in our era. This type of behaviour, if carried on for long
periods, can become a mental withdrawal, a controllable and
repetitive experience in which virtual reality is more highly esteemed
than relational life because it allows frustrations to be avoided and
pleasure to be enjoyed in a deceptively gratifying, parallel, sensory
world.

In this chapter, I explore the pathological dependence on the
Internet from the point of view of a psychic withdrawal.

The Internet can facilitate immersion into a fantasy world in which
one is not alone, since this form of unreality can be shared with others;
withdrawal into the Internet is a pleasurable exercise where, in a newly
created reality, an individual can live experiences in which he can do
absolutely whatever he wants. This is why it creates a pathological

dependence that tends to progressively ensnare people ready to be seduced by an imaginary world.

An example of this type of dependence is forty-year-old Attilio, a high-ranking manager in an international company, who comes to a consultation to seek a cure. I learn from the patient that he turned to me after his wife had threatened to leave him. For a number of years, he has lived two parallel lives: in the first, he is a loving husband who highly esteems his wife and much appreciates her beauty; in the second, which runs parallel to the first, he devotes himself to the Internet, spending hours online every day in chat rooms looking for women to have virtual relationships with, which sometimes lead to real encounters. Attilio says he has no intention of betraying his wife, whom he loves and with whom he hopes to have children, but he has been increasingly captivated by this space in which he can conquer unknown people who promise boundless experiences. Lately, the length of time he has spent online has further increased, to the extent of making his wife suspicious; she discovered all his secret contacts, felt betrayed, and decided to leave him. The patient is truly worried by this; he wants to cure himself, but, at the same time, would like someone to explain to his wife that his escape into the virtual world is far from a real betrayal.

A personal experience

Shortly after my book *The Sadomasochistic Perversion: The Entity and the Theories* (2003) (first published in Italian in 1999) was published, an acquaintance told me that my name was appearing on many Internet sites. For a moment, I was struck by the idea of having become suddenly famous; I thought my book must have been received unexpectedly well and went to have a look online.

Naturally, the sites that hosted comments about my book were not the highly respected sites I had hoped to find; instead, to my great surprise, they were sadomasochistic sites. Some of these included very attentive and detailed reviews of my book. The comments were not favourable: my text was a boring exercise by an amateur professor who pretended to understand the practice of sadomasochism, refusing to acknowledge its beneficial aspects and analysing its dangers. The comments were highly sarcastic. In that moment, I fully realised the existence of the extensive and invisible network of the web that, in the anonymous space of the Internet, weaves relationships, forms opinions, and attracts followers—also to sadomasochism.

Some comments claimed that the presence of sadomasochistic sites on the web is by no means a negative thing; it performs a beneficial action of containing, thus avoiding the more extreme tendencies of this sexual inclination. It seemed to me that the authors of these comments had posed a question that I had not sufficiently considered: are these sites (all sorts exist, for fetishists, sadomasochists, transvestites, paedophiles, and so on) tantamount to a transitional space with a containing function or are they a means for consolidating perverse practices and, perhaps, even augmenting them?

The Internet

The Internet is a system of networks, open to everyone, that defies any oligarchic or authoritarian type of arrangement; it is a new communicative democracy opposed to any type of censure.

The Internet can satisfy the desire for relationships but, paradoxically, it can increase solitude and become an enclosed place. Let us consider, for example, the difference that exists between one adolescent who uses the computer as a tool for knowledge and creativity and another who is passively engulfed by simulation games or porn sites.

The Internet is also an area of games played by the collective imagination, as, for example, the simulation game *SimCity*, in which the player becomes mayor of a city and decides how to regulate life there by making town-planning, financial, and work decisions.

More than a video game, *Second Life* is also a real simulation of life, an alternative life; you can project your alter ego into this imaginary space where it will live in a virtual three-dimensional world.

Virtual reality

The term *virtual reality* is much bandied about nowadays, but it implies a contradiction: if the noun *reality* relates to what is certain, verifiable, and existing, the adjective *virtual* refers to what is imaginary and hypothetical.

Virtual reality is present in many of our beliefs; it is enough that they are shared. For example, who among us would not be able to describe Father Christmas, a character present not only in the psychic reality of children but also in the memories of adults? Who among us has never heard of Donald Duck? Both Father Christmas and Donald Duck exist in the world of the imagination, in short, the virtual world. We are surprised only if someone says he has met and talked to Father Christmas and Donald Duck. In this case, Donald Duck is no longer the funny bumbling character who metaphorically alludes to aspects that can be found in all of us, but has become a real perception deprived of every symbolic meaning.

Many narratives created by man—for example, myths—have their origins in the imagination and maintain a virtual existence. Many ideal constructions that bind together peoples and nations, perhaps even religions, can be considered virtual realities. They remain valid because they have been consolidated by authority and the contribution of creative spirits, and they represent shared values.

So, what is the specific nature of the virtual reality on the Internet?

Silvio Merciai (2002) has assembled numerous opinions of psychologists, psychiatrists, and psychoanalysts about why and how people use the Internet. Some of them think the new digital reality represents a significant expansion of our perceptive horizon, a sort of Copernican revolution of our multiple selves. More modestly, others point out its regressive and manipulative limits.

If we want to optimise the first point of view, we could say that virtual reality is a powerful tool of knowledge that allows an intuitive, unconscious, almost childlike approach to the perception of a phenomenon. With such a tool, it is possible to create simulated contexts in which we can move around and interact; it is possible to represent phenomena that we cannot see but we can represent in an imagined dimension. In the scientific world, to take the field of physics, this opportunity is extremely useful.

Virtual reality can also be created with tools that realise the perception of *being inside*, objects that are called "immersive": a helmet, a pair of glasses, and so on.

Some neuroscientists have carried out experiments aimed at exchanging identities among people. An article in *The New York Times* (1 December 2008) describes the possibility of creating the real illusion of *being in another person's body* and reports the technique of Henrik

Ehrsson of the Karolinska Institute in Stockholm (Carey, 2008). A person stands in front of the researcher; both wear headgear with special glasses, and touch each other with their hands. The neuro-scientist has small video cameras that explore the environment; the volunteer's glasses are connected to these and so he sees everything that the researcher sees. The individual then begins to "perceive himself" as belonging to the body of the other; in a few seconds, the transformation is complete. The experiment shows that, when misled by sensory and optical stimuli, the mind can adopt another identity as though it were its own. Neuroscientists believe that the brain can be easily misled because it spends its entire life inside a body; since the eyes are perceived as positioned in the cranium, that is, in the person, the individual believes he is what his eyes see.

These are just a few of the many aspects that allow us to under-stand how virtual reality can enlarge our explorative horizon.

On the other hand, the words of Baudrillard (1999) help us reflect on the regressive aspect of using the Internet:

> . . . everything that exists in the real is positioned inside a differenti-ated universe, whereas the virtual is an integrated universe . . . in virtual reality everything is in effect possible, but the position of the subject is dangerously threatened, if not eliminated.

In short, Baudrillard believes that the virtual can absorb the real and that the distinction between subject and object no longer exists in the virtual dimension.

Lemma (2010) points out that the Internet's virtual space chal-lenges history, the individual's transitory nature, and even the percep-tion of his body. Every difference between individuals is abolished through imitative identifications. Consequently, the differences between the internal and the external world and between what is and what is fantasied disappear. Multiple identities can be quickly adopted and equally rapidly discarded; in this way, many "floating identities" (Raulet, 1991) that cannot be integrated and that remain split from each other are created.

Towards unreality

In previous chapters, I have already pointed out how some psycho-pathological experiences in the adult derive from a *withdrawal into sensory fantasy*, which is configured from childhood as the creation of a dissociated reality. It is important to distinguish this dissociated reality in which the child lives from other forms of the imagination, such as playing or dreamt illusions.

It is necessary to understand what game is played in using the Internet: the childhood game aimed at creating a space for the imagination or one that wants to construct a dissociated mental area, full of made-up figures that are treated as real. It is possible to grasp the transition from playful to pathological use when the fiction is no longer regarded as such but becomes a real sensory reality that distances the individual from the real symbolic world. This new sensory dimension ensnares the individual, who loses his capacity to maintain contact with his psychic reality and to perceive himself as emotionally linked to other human beings.

During the 1980s, Japan was gripped by the phenomenon of the *otakus*, groups of adolescents immersed in virtual reality and in love with the heroines of video games and television idols; some of them lived quite cut off from all reality (Vallario, 2008). Today, these young Japanese auto-recluses, slaves to the Internet (called *hihikomori*), number more than one million: one per cent of the population and two per cent of adolescents.

Internet pathology

Carrara and Zanda (2008) recall that the first person to talk about psychopathology deriving from the Internet was the American psychiatrist Ivan Goldberg, in 1995, who identified "Internet addiction disorder" and immediately put it up online for the public's attention. All traces of this discussion have been lost. Goldberg's diagnostic criteria followed those for disorders of drug addiction and included symptoms of abstinence and reduced attention span as negative consequences of the behaviour in question.

Some years later, the American psychiatrist Kimberley Young (1998) gave scientific dignity (this time in esteemed journals) to a series of clinical cases that she called "Internet addictions", or pathological dependence on the Internet, dividing them into various types, with "cybersexual addiction" taking the lead position in her classification.

Cybersex

The Internet has obviously made its way into psychopathology, too, especially in the realm of sexuality.

Virtual sex, or *cybersex* are the names given to the use of new technologies for acquiring material that stimulates sexual fantasies. These new ways of sexual gratification take on a variety of forms: the pornography of the Internet, chat lines on the phone, or private sexual communications. All these activities are called *virtual* because they are based on the capacity to create imaginary scenes that include other actors. In fact, the person remains alone and the sexual act consists of masturbation; the adjective *virtual* refers to the fact that the scene created by technological means corresponds to, or stimulates, the personal fantasies of the individual making use of it. Studies undertaken in the USA (Cooper, 2002) tell us that at least seventy per cent of what is spent online is for the acquisition of virtual sex. In numerous cases, we are seeing a true toxicophiliac dependence on the Internet.

To give an idea of the dimension of the phenomenon in Italy, I would like to report some statistics (Fabbri, 2006).

It seems that 5.6% of Internet users spend between eleven and twenty-five hours a week online looking for pornographic material, while eleven per cent of these users suffer from a serious dependence and are online for up to forty-five hours a week. Sex ranks third in the web's overall economy. Twelve per cent of all sites is a pornography site, as is twenty-five per cent of requests to search engines and thirty-five per cent of all downloads. Every second, almost thirty thousand people surf a porn site, and every day 266 new porn sites are created.

Within this phenomenon, it seems that men and women have different ways of behaving: while men mainly surf porn sites and download images for voyeuristic arousal, women are more interested in erotic experiences based on language and so turn to chat lines where they can improvise relationships that have an imagined or exhibitionist component, but which sometimes conclude in a real meeting.

Recently, new techniques have been invented for making virtual sex more satisfying. Until this point, it was possible to enjoy only a voyeuristic arousal through assisting at the sexual exploits of one's own alter ego; now, there is an interactive suit that lets you physically feel the sensations experienced by your own character. In practice, if the character receives a caress, the individual seated in front of the screen receives and feels on his own body the sensation of being caressed. So, we are on the threshold of a technological operation that allows enjoyment of what Freud had prophesied as the most primitive and regressed level of the libido, *auto-erotism*. In theory, it will be possible to create with the imagination an auto-erotic withdrawal that completely disregards any relational investment with real, living people.

I shall now explore in greater depth the kind of mind that is ensnared by the net.

A patient

This material refers to the analysis of Fausta, described in Chapter Nine. I present it here to show how the delusional story acted out in the transference can find its continuation in the web.

> "Voilà Valentino (but is that your real name? It's not important, I like the name). Seeing that it's almost your saint's day, seeing that you like to read and write, and seeing that you like surprises and new ideas . . . let's play a little.
>
> You write, "This girl, if I could only look into her eyes right now . . . I would take hold of her hands and sure . . . in the reflections of the flames sparkling in the fireplace in the study of my house where she is with me . . . I would see her sweet face redden . . . I would kiss her slowly, gently . . . and then suddenly embrace her, pulling her strongly to me . . ."
>
> I write, "I feel your arms holding me. Your hot breath in my left ear sets my hormones on fire so that they course excitedly through my body filling me with desire and memories of other arms holding me, hands caressing me, mouths kissing me, moments, the most beautiful, of ecstasy, of orgasms and of perdition . . ."

This is the beginning of an online dialogue between Fausta and an unknown man. It is a typewritten text that faithfully reports the long exchange between the two and that was given to the analyst at the end of a session. Written by both of them, but always in the first person as a dialogue between two lovers, the story is the faithful account of their communication over days and days; it goes on for ten pages, full of exciting erotic details, and lingers on the most detailed description of the sensations of two bodies being reciprocally penetrated and repeatedly reaching the peak of total orgasm.

Fausta confesses to the analyst that the past days had been incredibly arousing for her; her day revolved around the moment when she could click open her inbox and resume communication with this mysterious and fascinating interlocutor. She also says that in certain moments she was thinking of meeting him but, in the end, when he actually proposed this, she said no and the whole experience evaporated. The analyst listens with puzzlement to this communication and wonders what escaped him in the relationship with the patient, who, in recent months, had seemed to him to be more integrated and capable of affective dependence.

What does it mean for her to have reached a virtual orgasm?

The analyst was convinced that, after the work accomplished in their sessions, the risk of erotic flight on Fausta's part was negligible. Yet, it did not happen like that: her flight into sexual fantasy took off once more, apparently disregarding the transference. Naturally, the analyst thinks that in offering him the text the patient was still trying to arouse his voyeurism and, possibly, even inviting him to have sexual relations with her.

I have taken up Fausta's analytic story once again to show how, in her case, sexual flight into the Internet represented nothing but the progression of the analytic events, of the erotic transference, and of the flight into an illusory world. It is as though Fausta had found on the Internet the pleasure of arousing and being aroused that had been denied her in the relationship with the therapist after analysis of the erotic transference, which had been worked on during the previous months.

Withdrawal into fantasy

Withdrawal into sensory fantasy continues for a long time alongside the relational world, with the two worlds never meeting. Virtual reality is highly prized because it allows the frustrations of real life to be worked out. This function is often carried out by the Internet, as it allows the projection of pleasure in a virtual world that is constituted as an enclosed, controllable, and repetitive experience.

*   *   *

Ermanno is a young man of twenty-two who came to me to begin an analysis. He looks as though he is suffering greatly; his face is pallid and emaciated. He speaks in a soft, low voice and says he has no friends and that he lives within the narrow limits of his family—his mother and sister. The only activity that allows him to have any social relationships is through being creative. He says he is good at modelling clay and succeeds in expressing this skill in the groups of children who attend the parish church activities. A paternal aunt was important during his childhood, an authoritarian woman devoted to a world of religious sacrifice, who replaced not only his mother—silent and depressed—but also his father, who died prematurely when the patient was ten.

Ermanno has always had a delicate appearance and has never been fond of the sporting activities that would have helped his relationships with boys of his own age. When he was an adolescent, he often felt he was an object of their derision; he did not know how to defend himself from them or make friends with them.

It certainly seems as though he suffered a block in his emotional development. Having arrived at adulthood, he feels very disorientated; he says he repeats the same dreams in which he is out in the open, or in deserted or unkempt landscapes, with no human presence at all.

It is not clear whether Ermanno has ever had any sexual experiences. He is reticent about this and seems almost to have banished any desire in that direction from his mind. Then, very hesitatingly, he talks about the erotic fantasies he had in high school; he remembers that he was attracted to boys that were good-looking and vigorous. He dreamt of being able to merge with them and their attractiveness, but he felt himself to be so ugly and contemptible. He never succeeded in having a homosexual experience, but he devised a strategy that is possible to realise thanks to the Internet: he took part in the chat lines. There, it was possible to disguise himself and to present himself as a woman. So began a hugely exciting game. Online, he could live as a woman and have the power of seducing men, of being the object of their desires, of their ardent communications and demands.

Ermanno says that after a while the game was no longer amusing; on the contrary, he now feels the desire to have a real human relationship. Unfortunately, he feels completely lacking in the wherewithal to make this happen.

* * *

Transitional space

We may suppose that a flight into the virtual space of the Internet might, for some patients, be a defensive flight, a sort of transitional space where fantasies can flow freely without control and where it is possible to hide, but from where it is also possible to exit gradually whenever you want.

I do not know if this hypothesis can be applied to all patients who live "in the computer" because, in my view, there is a conceptual difference between the *transitional area* and the *psychic withdrawal*. The difference is one of quality, not quantity. The transitional area is an open space in which the illusion plays a primary role because the child, though not yet able to create symbols, is on the way to doing so. The transitional object traces a developmental path, albeit in a dimension of non-differentiation between the *me* and the *not-me*. In psychic withdrawal, completely occupied by the sensory experience, there is no potential space for development; the allusive and symbolic experience is erased. On the Internet, pleasure derives from the fact that the objects are predictable and controllable, and not complex and contradictory like real emotional relations.

In the solitary imagination (created and enjoyed by the patient) a simple click can evoke bodies, and stimuli necessary to arousal, with which one can do whatever one wants. Furthermore, it is possible, with one's eyes, to take for oneself the exciting qualities of the object.

Psychic withdrawal is not a suspended area between fantasy and reality: instead, it is a psychopathological construction that exercises a hypnotic attraction over the rest of the personality, which is, consequently, continually impoverished. Observation of people who fall into this trap clearly shows that they reach a true state of regression typical of an addicted nature.

The Internet does not, in itself, create the pathology, but it is the ideal means for bringing it to light when the premises for it exist.

A stimulus for perversion?

The question posed at the start of this chapter—whether a voyeuristic use of the Internet limits the perverse act to the virtual world, thus avoiding the risk of acting it out in reality—remains a controversial point. On the one hand, the pornographic site lends itself to functioning as a container of the perversion, whereas, on the other, compulsive consultation of the site enables the perverse construction to spread and confirms the validity of the delusional nucleus that sustains it.

I do not believe that a pornographic site can mitigate highly destructive perversions. The fact that the Marquis de Sade wrote books instead of continuing to act out his perverse fantasies does not stem from the containing function of writing, but from the fact that he was materially deprived of his freedom through being imprisoned; previously, when free in his castle, he had begun to employ young servants of both sexes with the aim of using them for a complex act of sexual abuse and bodily mortification, which was to culminate in a criminal orgy. Sade could not carry out his plan because he was denounced and imprisoned in the Bastille, where, unable to act out his fantasies, he began to write the novels that were to make him famous.

The Internet is the frame, the imaginative field, into which every virtual representation of the perverse sexual panorama can be projected and, therefore, not acted out in reality; however, often, it is also a path that fosters the progression of the pathological process.

Regarding this point, in an article devoted to the risks run by the technological child, Amati-Mehler (1984) notes,

> The supremacy of images relates back to a primitive function of the mind, when visual thought prevailed. This is an interesting point worthy of further research because it implies a certain "hypnotic" and addictive effect that makes it difficult to set boundaries between self and the game and that invades the whole of psychic functioning, sometimes for hours on end. In my opinion, this aspect merits further attention because it facilitates regression to states of undifferentiation between oneself and what is outside oneself. (p. 302)

Describing himself in *The Tears of Eros*, Bataille (2001[1961]) gives us an extraordinarily eloquent example of the importance of the visual image in triggering the perverse climax. One of the ways he reached sexual ecstasy was by identifying himself completely with a young Chinese man photographed as he was dying after being horribly tortured. The cruel image, the ecstatic gaze, the flayed ribs of the dying man caused Bataille convulsions of pleasure. Bataille identifies with the prisoner and relates that during sexual ecstasy a flash of light passed through his head from bottom to top, as voluptuous as the passage of the seed during sex. He says he felt himself transformed into an erect phallus and thinks that ecstasy (religious) and the mental orgasm of the perverse act have much in common. The photograph used by Bataille to reach ecstasy (a significant detail: the image was given to him by his analyst) is nothing compared to the myriad figures of the perverse imagination that today's Internet world makes available.

As therapists, we are called on to deal with this boundless virtual sphere by our patients, who use it and fuel it, astounding us with the immense, invisible, and silent network that surrounds us and whose importance in psychopathology we must increasingly recognise.

CHAPTER FIFTEEN

Some problems in treating borderline patients

"... ruleless fantasy approaches madness, where fantasy plays completely with the human being and the unfortunate victim has not control at all over the course of his representations"

(Kant, 2006[1798], p. 75)

There are many reasons why the treatment of borderline patients is difficult. I will explore two of them in this chapter. First, these patients are unable to understand their own psychic functioning and the reasons for others' behaviours due to their lack of an emotional–receptive capacity. Second, since they come from a traumatic environment, they are particularly susceptible to frustrations and react violently to conflict, attempting vindictive revenge against the objects they clash with. This is why borderline patients often perpetuate a very tenacious bond with their traumatising primary objects, from which they cannot separate.

As is known, the term "borderline" was first used to define a psychopathological syndrome halfway between neurosis and psychosis, characterised by a group of symptoms that belonged to both nosographic categories but which implied potential psychotic development concealed behind a neurotic façade.

This nosological category was only isolated as a clinical and diagnostic entity in its own right, with its own particular characteristics, in the 1960s. Kernberg (1967) was the first to endow it with the statute of a *stable and specific pathological organisation* of the personality based on laws of its own functioning, describing four characteristics specific to this structure:

- a weak ego: incapacity to contain anxiety, lack of control over impulses, lack of development of sublimatory functions;
- regression towards the primary thought process;
- specific defence mechanisms: splitting, primitive idealisation, projective identification, denial, omnipotence, and object devaluation;
- pathological internalised object relations.

A natural function

Development of the analytic process is fraught with difficulty with borderline patients; the conditions allowing the analytic process to develop are very complex because they cannot make use of an unconscious emotional–receptive apparatus that allows them to perceive their own emotional state and to monitor their behaviour with others (Fonagy & Target, 1996). These deficiencies would seem to originate from a series of infantile emotional traumas resulting from parental figures responding to the child's normal turbulence with aggressive rejections.

Research on the childhood of these patients reveals that they suffered a high number of emotional traumas and early abandonments (Adler, 1988).

Generally, parents were found to be incapable of being a supportive object for the emotional growth of their children; they were distant or intrusive with a tendency to use their children as an extension of themselves. In particular, their behaviour was changeable and unpredictable, so that they were experienced as confusing and untrustworthy. Even though cases of early abandonment or sexual abuse have been recorded, the constant common element is the lack of emotional contact throughout the whole growing period.

These childhood experiences produce a keen sensitivity and intolerance towards frustrations, even those that are inevitable. It seems that borderline patients remain prisoners of the effects that the emotional trauma produced on their psyche for the whole of their lives, as though they were governed by a continuous manic reparation of the damage suffered.

Precisely because they lack the capacity for emotive understanding, their behaviour is repetitive, impulsive, and aggressive, directed towards negating the tension rather than towards understanding the reasons behind conflict in human relationships.

These introductory remarks concur with what Fonagy emphasised on a number of occasions: borderline patients present a deficit in the reflective function caused by a deficient maternal response to the child's need for mirroring and, in particular, an insufficient degree of coherence and security of the early object relations.

Acquisition of the reflective function is part of a developmental trend that starts from the affective resonance in the first months of life, as described by Stern (1985), passes through responding to the mood of the other in babies of eight months, up to understanding the others' intentions as demonstrated in games of cooperation by babies of fourteen months. More advanced knowledge of one's own and others' mental states is acquired at about four years of age.

The reflective function, therefore, is not innate, but is acquired during growth and continues to develop in subsequent years.

As I have attempted to explain in Chapter Seven, the deficit in emotive comprehension inherent in the borderline pathology depends on the fact that the traumatic experiences occurred in the period in which the apparatuses responsible for the development of unconscious emotional–receptive functions were being formed. Difficult childhood experiences encourage the construction of pathological structures that compromise the construction of the function that governs unconscious intrapsychic communication.

This is why one could talk of borderline patients as being subjects without an unconscious, or, rather, with an inadequate emotional–receptive unconscious, whose most common characteristic is the compromising of interpersonal relationships inside and outside the transference. Preserving bonds or maintaining a stable identity seems impossible for them, or dangerous: they oscillate between an extreme need for dependence and the risk of feeling themselves enclosed and confined. This has led some analysts to propose special forms of therapy that bear in mind the instability of these patients. To cite one as an example of all, I would like to mention Kernberg's transference focused psychotherapy (TFP) (2010): his underlying proposition is that the therapist—aiming to lessen the actings out outside the analysis—should provide interpretations focused exclusively on the transference, while the patient is followed by a team that assists and contains him. In the transference, the inconsistent emotional dyads that are not integrated into the rest of the personality would be focused on and could, in this way, be worked through.

In this chapter, I highlight an element that, in my view, can always be found in the borderline pathology, and that is the tendency to maintain a type of sadomasochistic bond with the original frustrating objects.

The relationships of these patients are partial, chaotic, but often very intense. They manifest a high degree of personal hypersensitivity, confusion about their own identity, conflicting emotional responses, and difficulty in behaving in a coherent and organised way.

A high level of instability and unpredictability is the main characteristic; this aspect also emerges during therapy, characterised by turbulent progress marked by repetitive impulsive acts, suicidal or self-mutilating tendencies, or moments of intense dependence alternating with estrangement or interruptions.

A patient

I will describe only the beginning of the psychoanalytic therapy of this patient[18] in order to highlight how the characteristics of the borderline organisation are represented as early as in embryonic form.

> Emma, a nice, sporty-looking blonde woman, is a successful journalist. She looks as though she has had to struggle quite a bit in life and appears traumatised and depressed.
>
> "I've been depressed since my life began; I am tormented by anxiety and nightmares. I had a complete breakdown when my stepmother let me down again last spring. I can't live without medicines [she takes antidepressants and sleeping pills and has a drink problem]. I can't stop this absurd behaviour. I'm frightened my marriage has broken down."

Later on, she confesses that when she cannot manage the tension, she goes to a club where people take part in group sex. She has constant clashes with her husband and they are both argumentative. Her latest crisis was triggered by her stepmother's behaviour, which led to a violent argument. Although Emma says she does not love her, she still seems very dependent on her and the inevitable conflicts leave devastating effects.

Emma's mother died when she was a year old after sepsis set in following a routine operation; at that time she was depressed because of the death of her mother. An elderly great-aunt took care of her until she was four: she remembers loving this woman very much.

When her father married for the second time, Emma, to her great disappointment, had to return home. Soon, two half-brothers were born.

From then on, her life became terrible: she was hit by her stepmother almost every day, often without reason. She remembers receiving a terrible blow to her face from her father. When she started going to school, her stepmother authorised her teachers to hit her if she was not obedient. At home, her parents behaved violently to each other; once her stepmother threw a bottle of beer at her drunk father's head and the house was full of blood. She was no longer allowed to see her great-aunt, who did not remain living nearby but moved to another town.

Emma was an intelligent student and got her degree with ease. Her first marriage ended in divorce and the daughter born from it lives with her. She married a second time eight years ago, to a good-looking Greek journalist who behaves in a very macho way. There is a lot of violence and huge clashes between them. Her husband is a not very successful journalist and does not earn a lot of money; he is very egocentric.

Emma has always been a brilliant journalist, more highly esteemed than her husband, but their conflicts have interfered with her career. She is currently experiencing a moment of professional crisis. When she is fifty, she has the right to a permanent position, but the directors of the radio station where she has been working for the past eleven years are attempting to get rid of her, as they do with all the other older colleagues.

She reports two dreams in the first two sessions of analysis.

"I am going towards the parish church with my husband. The church doesn't look like it does really. Two lances are hanging from high above in the central nave, in the corridor between the pews. I'm saying something to my husband that he doesn't understand; something along the lines of those lances are too much for me to bear. On the left a christening is being held and so I'm speaking in a whisper. I don't want to disturb them. My husband moves ahead and I follow him towards the altar. There is a woman preparing something who greets me: 'How nice you've still come to visit us'. Suddenly my parents (my father and stepmother) appear in front of me; my nose runs but I don't have any handkerchiefs so I wipe it with my hand. My father looks disgusted. My mother, wearing boots of snakeskin, lifts her foot and tries to kick me in the stomach. I grab her boot, slide it off and hit her. I do it out of self-defence."

She explains that her brother is expecting his second child.

Then she relates a second dream of the same night. "In the dream there was a room filled with demons, living things and lianas. A heart was removed from the graveyard and put inside a plastic bag in my husband's jacket. It smelt horribly. I was saying, 'It's got to go!'"

These two dreams, related at the start of the analysis, seem especially important because they describe very accurately the traumatic experience, the way the patient reacts to it, and the state of her internal objects. The church where she was with her husband is not a calm place of prayer, but a place full of potential violence with weapons hanging from the ceiling. The sadomasochistic relationship with her stepmother is clearly portrayed in the dream. Certainly, the patient is attacked first (both by her father, who expresses disgust for her lack of decorum, and by her stepmother), but her response is equally blindly violent.

Before the clash in the dream with her parents there was a moment of tranquillity when a woman said how nice it was to see her again. It seems as though Emma had been able to recover for a brief moment in the dream a positive experience with a female figure that must certainly be linked to her earliest years spent in her great-aunt's house. However, the positive moment lasts for a very short time and is brusquely shattered by the violent outburst with her stepmother.

The first dream seems to repeat a very real and actual experience. Even though her stepmother has displayed malice towards her from early infancy (Emma recalls that when her stepmother and father went on holiday with her two younger siblings, she was left with the neighbours), she has never been able to separate psychologically from her and preserves a type of sadomasochistic, victimised bond with her. Any slight frustration provoked by the stepmother is sufficient to trigger infinite pain and revengeful anger.

The second dream seems even more significant. The atmosphere is most unsettling, with a decomposing heart that must be got rid of. In this case, it could refer to the patient's heart or to the heart of her love objects: her dead mother or her husband, with whom she is now on a collision course. In the dream, it seems as though she herself has to kill her sensitive and affective part in order to eliminate any hope of reparation. In confirmation of this, she remembers that when she was six she often vomited; she suffered profound states of anguish and missed her mother terribly. On one occasion she went to the graveyard and lay down on her tomb: "It was cold and so felt good."

It would appear that this childhood experience was crucial for laying the foundations for her way of cutting adrift her affective part, thus becoming devoid of emotional contact, in a state of unconscious fusion with her dead mother.

As is typical of the therapies of borderline patients, Emma's analysis progressed through alternating highs and lows and extreme situations.

The scene was dominated in the first period by promiscuous sexual relationships with men contacted on the Internet, a manic type of behaving with the acquisition of costly domestic pets, and a lifestyle way beyond her income.

The worst conflictual situations were with her love objects, first of all her husband, from whom she succeeded in separating, and then with her daughter, who developed risky behaviours in adolescence. The tension with the management of the radio station where she worked was no less serious; in threatening to sack her, they annulled her as a person and as a professional figure.

There were also some extremely risky moments: crises of depression, the desire to end it all, and a constant feeling of the futility of the therapy, in spite of a very tenacious analytic bond. The events of the transference were certainly less significant when compared to the complexity of the extra-transference relationships and conflicts, but all of this led to difficult countertransferal moments, due to the patient's skill in involving the analyst, too, into the events of her life.

As in all borderline conditions, it was necessary in this case, too, to sustain the analytic relationship on the basis of the positive experience that the patient had had with a good parental figure, the great-aunt, and protect her from the storms of the conflict as represented in the first dream with the stepmother.

Maintaining a balanced position in the countertransference between participation and the correct level of distance is a complex task in our relationship with borderline patients. The analyst must know how to keep a good balance, even if this is by no means easy. Despite all the attempts by the patient to totally involve the analyst in his life outside analysis, the analyst must, at all costs, avoid colluding with the patient's implicit and explicit requests.

Rosenfeld (1978) makes a very useful observation regarding this when he says that borderline patients differ from psychotics because they project their omnipotent narcissistic structure into situations of reality that "conceal" it, since these situations function in an objectively analogous way to their pathogenic structures.

The sadomasochistic bond

While it is true that the suffering of these patients is rooted in an early narcissistic wound, it is also true that the whole borderline organisation is directed towards vengeful revenge for wrongs suffered, past and present.

This is why borderline patients maintain a very tenacious bond with their primary traumatising objects, from which they are unable to separate; they never reach a state of true mourning, that is, they can never pardon the traumatising objects of the past or accept that they can never regain what they have lost.

During conflicts that cause the old traumas to re-emerge, these patients end up fighting against the frustrating object in a never-ending battle that will lead them to be violent against themselves, too.

*   *   *

Carla is a seriously disordered patient. Since early childhood, she has suffered from anorexic episodes. The first trauma ensued from a pyloric dysfunction in her fist months of life which caused feeding problems that took the family some time to recognise (they thought she was just being capricious).

During adolescence, the patient was admitted to hospital a number of times for serious anorexic episodes and various attempts were made to place her in a community in order to distance her from the family context, worsened by constant conflict with her mother. Despite everything, Carla went on to get married and have children. Her relationship with people dear to her is always precarious, bordering on catastrophe, with suicidal threats and gestures that lead to further hospital admissions. Her ample symptomatology includes panic attacks and periods of anorexia alternated with bulimic orgies. Furthermore, even though she is over forty, has had children and created a family, she is still linked to her mother by a sadomasochistic bond. For example, if her mother leaves town to visit her sister or for a short holiday, Carla develops worrying symptoms on an eating and behavioural level. Her last hospitalisation after a medicine-induced suicide attempt is extremely recent.

Returning to analysis, she tells me that her self-harming gesture was caused by a profound misunderstanding with her husband and by the fact that she, as usual, does not know how to manage conflict except by self-destructive behaviour.

The calm after this storm lasted only a couple of days: the sessions are immediately full of threats and declarations of violence; she wants to throw herself out of the window or gorge on pills again. She has gone back to getting up very early in the morning in order to run furiously for an hour and arrives at the sessions breathless from cycling here when she could easily take public transport. In this way, she has managed to lose the small amount of weight gained that made her gauntness less unsettling. She does not sleep, she feels depressed, and fantasises about committing suicide. She adds that she has violent impulses against her children, who are her only love objects; for this reason she wants to be hospitalised. I tell her that her self-destructive tendency has once again unleashed itself. She seems surprised, but then admits that she is angry with her husband again, who has distanced himself from her, and hates her mother, who feigns indifference. She says she is fascinated by the idea of hospitalisation: a place to find refuge in, a uterus to which she could blissfully return.

*   *   *

What happens in Carla's psyche? She does not have a space of her own; to survive she has to remain indissolubly bound to her objects (mother, husband, and analyst). The old sadomasochistic bond, which had caused her serious anorexic symptomatology during adolescence, is still active and reappears at every frustration, far removed from awareness.

The attack on the object is not expressed with vital anger, but with self-destruction. Like a suicide terrorist, Carla hurls her body against

the hated object in order to strike it and involve it in her self-destruction. Carla's trigger towards self-annihilation is the response that
bound her to the traumatic object in a reciprocally destructive thrust;
anorexia is, in fact, a psychic strategy towards self-annihilation that
involves a violent attack against the bodily self and against the frustrating object, in a never-ending sequence.

In particular, the borderline patient shows an incapacity to tolerate
frustration, both those that are inevitable and those caused by a
malevolent object, to which he reacts with vindictive behaviour
directed towards annihilating the adversary or with a destructive
attack on himself. Patent narcissistic susceptibility, probably matured
in some privileged infant relationship, renders the borderline patient
both fragile and overbearing. This pushes him to a victimistic use of
the trauma and to the use of anger as an exciting element.

The analyst's attention in the relationship with the patient must be
directed at avoiding entering into the vicious sadomasochistic circle,
knowing how to grade his interventions, tuning them to the patient's
receptive capacity, and understanding moment by moment.

What I have said so far accounts for only a part of the complex
mental condition of the borderline patient. Bearing in mind what I
wrote in Chapter Five on the construction of the withdrawal, I believe
we can say that this type of patient often lives in a world of illusionary and falsified fantasies.

When this illusionary world is threatened by frustration or
attacked by reality, then never-ending anger is unleashed against the
self and against whoever is perceived as being responsible for the failure. In other words, it is a reaction to a narcissistic wound, a threat to
the patient's grandiosity, which, paradoxically, also fuels his vitality.

When the crisis is unleashed, it is also important to foresee any
possible self-harming actions which could put the patient's life in
danger. In these cases, a superego is unleashed that attacks the patient
with brutal force, punishing him for his failures and involving
whoever seems to be at the origin of the frustration in the vindictive
action.

*   *   *

A twenty-five-year-old patient of mine, who lived in a fantasy world,
had spent her first analytic sessions often showing me drawings or
other "creations" she had made, whose contents I limited myself to

interpreting. Her implicit aim was to convince me that I had in therapy a great artist destined for immediate success. Another characteristic aspect of this woman was to arrive at the session, usually late, dressed very carefully and often in clothes of times gone by, thus revealing that, in that moment, she was identified with a fantasy character. Neither was it easy to understand how much was real and how much was "dreamt" in her affective relationships. This was dramatically confirmed to me when her relationship with a partner, who lived in another city and with whom there was clearly a reciprocal illusory pact, was broken off by the latter. This was followed by a suicidal gesture.

But even before this occurred, I had been very struck by her dreams, which were exceptionally violent: in general, she was tortured by men who threatened to rape her, or who actually did so. I had come to think that perhaps she had been abused in her childhood, but progressively I realised that in the dream a brutal superego was represented that sprang into action whenever the patient, forced outside her illusionary (amorous or performative) world, had to face up to the inevitable narcissistic disappointment and frustration.

Hate in the countertransference

One of the reasons that makes therapy with borderline patients difficult is that they lack the capacity to contain and modulate their emotions. Lacking the capacity to understand their own emotional states—the principal instrument that enables emotions to be contained and transformed—means that it is not possible to prevent them from erupting in violent and overwhelming ways. It is also difficult to predict the transference: it can pass from moments of calmness and tranquillity to stormy and explosive passages.

This type of patient is very far from what is usually called the depressive position, which is the capacity to put oneself in the shoes of others, to understand their behaviour and limits; in particular, it does not allow another's suffering or their points of view to be understood.

Winnicott (1949) has described the hate felt by the analyst in the countertransference. With these patients who continually put us to the test, we cannot avoid feeling such an emotion: always late, the sessions missed, the abrupt mood swings, forgetting to pay, the constant attempt to involve the analyst and make him act out in the patient's stead, all this creates the sensation that we are relentlessly bombarded but have no opportunity to really participate in the analytic events. However, despite the constant state of turbulence, the analytic therapy does proceed and gradually the patient also becomes more capable of modulating his own emotivity and of finding a place in the external world that is useful for relational exchange.

It is most probable that the long work of emotional containing on the part of the analyst serves to filter the patient's excessive turbulence and aggression and helps him progressively to construct an internal world in which the objects can take on loving characteristics.

In this chapter, I have described a number of characteristics of the borderline syndrome. I would like to end by recalling the most crucial:

- the constant presence of trauma in childhood and adolescence;
- a victimistic use of the trauma;
- anger as an exciting mental state;
- an incapacity to tolerate a normal degree of frustration;
- the impossibility of acceding to the depressive position;
- stormy shifts in transference;
- the urge to make the analyst act out;
- the presence of a sadistic superego;
- incapacity to identify with the other;
- living mainly in a fantasy world.

CHAPTER SIXTEEN

Elements for the analytic therapy of psychotic patients

"The delusion springs from your very innards and this insight floods your mind"

(A psychotic patient in analysis)

I n this chapter, I describe the most common problems in the therapy of psychotic patients. One of the main difficulties is the tenacious obstinacy with which the psychotic state imposes itself and conquers the healthy part of the personality. I aim to illustrate briefly some of the specific elements that the analyst must know how to grasp and propose to the patient in order to wean him from the seductive power of the delusional world.

The problems encountered in the treatment of psychotic patients depend on many factors, one of which is certainly represented by the fact that it is impossible for the analyst to use the same therapy method as for the neurotic patient. Just as physicists cannot use classical physics to study the atom, so psychoanalysts cannot use the psychoanalytic methodology created to understand neuroses to approach the world of psychosis. This deters many colleagues from accepting into therapy a patient who suffers from this symptomatology.

When we encounter this type of patient, we must not undervalue the progressive nature of the psychotic process and we must immediately intuit the dangerous path the patient might take. In other words, we must know how the psychotic mind functions and what the risks of treatment are.

A specific characteristic of psychosis is that once the pathological change has occurred, it reveals itself to be obstinately tenacious, as though the mutation that has occurred has wiped out the pre-existing structure—just like a volcanic lava flow. This leads to bewilderment in the analyst's countertransference, as he sees that the healthy part of the patient has disappeared, with which, up to that point, he had thought he could interact. The psychotic state resembles a river in spate that needs embankments to contain it.

Unlike the past, today, the extreme peaks of the psychotic symptomatology can be lessened by psychopharmacological means and it is possible to intervene positively during the crisis. Consequently, the analyst who intends to treat psychotic patients should always work together with a psychiatrist. Usually, psychotic patients arrive already in psychopharmacological care, begun during hospitalisation; if this is not the case, it is necessary to make arrangements with the patient and send him to a psychiatrist colleague who can see him regularly. This is an indispensable preliminary step because, if psychiatric intervention becomes necessary during treatment, the invitation at that moment to go to a psychiatrist would sound to the patient's ears like a refusal on the analyst's part to take care of him. Naturally, it is important to choose a psychiatrist colleague who empathises with the analytic therapy and is extremely careful not to interfere with it.

The psychotic part at the helm

My model for understanding psychotic functioning is based on the contrast, highlighted by Bion (1957), between the healthy part and the psychotic part of the personality. This model is also useful for dealing with perversions, where we can differentiate the healthy part from the perverse part of the personality. In the case of perversions, however, the perverse part, while wielding power over the healthy part, maintains a certain equilibrium and the conquest never involves the whole personality. In the case of the psychoses, instead, the psychotic part not only dominates the healthy part, but progressively colonises it and engulfs it until it gets rid of it entirely. A further difference is that the psychotic individual performs a radical overturning of thought and of the rules that foster comprehension of human relations. This is a long-lasting process; it begins in childhood, generally remains hidden during adolescence, and openly manifests itself during early adult-hood. When the healthy part is completely conquered by the sick part, the crisis emerges, which, at times, requires hospitalisation and psychopharmacological treatment. The psychotic episode, moreover, is a traumatic and destructuring event that leaves profound traces and creates strong inhibitions and distortions of thought that continue operating for a long time, even when the crisis is exhausted. Generally speaking, it is, therefore, preferable to work with the patient before the crisis manifests itself and, in any case, in the presence of only one psychotic episode.

The model of the psychotic part and the healthy part advanced by Bion has an immediate effect on the way of working with psychotic patients. During the therapy it is important, on the one hand, to stim-ulate the patient to understand how the psychotic part conquers him, and, on the other, to activate perception of the danger he risks in letting himself be seduced. This aspect of the therapy is not easy to put into practice because the patient does not readily communicate the delusional construction to the analyst since, in his eyes, it is a plea-surable mental state at the service of his omnipotence. It is only after-wards, when the crisis is full-blown, that the analyst discovers the extent to which he was taken in by the patient.

The damage to the emotional unconscious and to the capacity to think, unleashing the crisis, prevents it from being ever truly trans-formed, even when it has been overcome from a clinical point of view. Generally, the crisis is dissociated and remains encysted in the psyche, where it will produce constant instability. This explains why every breakdown leaves behind a further defect.

Treatment difficulties

Freud described repression as the process whereby thoughts and emotions that are incompatible with the conscious are repressed, that is, transferred to the unconscious. Bion maintains that repression is a physiological process that enables the transformation of sensory perceptions into thoughts.

The difficulty in our analytic work with psychotic patients stems, in large part, from the fact that they cannot use emotional thought as we do. To work through emotions, we make a large part of our conscious perceptions unconscious. Unconsciously worked through in this way, events acquire meaning and are integrated into the whole sphere of personal emotional experience. Dreams offer testimony of this constant linking up and giving emotional meaning to what we have experienced. The repression processes that the dream makes use of are reversible and allow us to go back to the experienced emotional reality through association.

This operation is based on the workings of the dynamic unconscious (the system studied by Freud) that allows constant symbolising and oscillation (Bion's semi-permeable membrane) between waking perception and dream perception.

All this is either lacking or highly deficient in the psychotic patient, at least while he is dominated by the psychotic part; consequently, it is not possible to make use of the traditional analytic technique which, to increase processes of awareness, is based on free associations and on the interpretation of repressed contents.

The laws of unconscious thought—discovered by psychoanalysis—that are involved with the functioning of the *unconscious psychic reality* (with its mechanisms of repression, unconscious conflict, symbolic transformation, the stages of child sexuality, and so on) do not perform during the psychotic state.

Therefore, I believe that the traditional analytic categories of the dynamic unconscious do not allow us to fully comprehend the specific nature of the illness and the apparently bizarre and mysterious way in which it is expressed.

In the psychotic state, the patient uses his mind not for understanding the world, but for producing images and sensations. Hallucinations, indeed, result from the sensory use of the mind that generates perceptions from the same sensory channels.

The dream delusion

In psychosis, the dream, too, can be a psychopathological construction: contrary to what Freud wrote when he stated that the psychosis has all the characteristics of a dream, the psychosis is exactly the opposite of a dream. A psychotic patient's dream can be a delusion; indeed, a distinction must be made between a *dream thought* and a *dream delusion*.

The absence of emotional unconscious work prevents any encounter between the dreamer who dreams the dream and the dreamer who understands it, exactly as occurs with the delusion. This explains the obscurity and incomprehensibility of some dreams of the psychotic state and the extreme difficulty that patient and analyst have in understanding them.

Despite this, dreams are still extremely useful since, as I explain further on, they represent a means of direct access to the psychotic transformation because this is described by them; occasionally, when the patient keeps his psychopathological construction secret, they are the only means available for exploring his propensity to be delusional. Then the analyst's capacity to grasp any traces of this transformation in the dream becomes absolutely crucial.

Some dreams predict the psychotic explosion, which can be caught by the ear of an analyst experienced in the therapy of such patients. An example is the dream manifested at the beginning of the delusional affair of President Schreber. I will give some examples of this type of dream in the chapters that follow.

The cancerous metastasis

As I have already stated, the explosion of a psychotic crisis leaves indelible traces and entails a complex work of reconstruction. It must not be forgotten that, once the crisis has occurred, the psychotic nucleus remains like a tree whose trunk has been felled but whose roots are well grounded in the earth.

This is why it would be much more effective to work in childhood or during adolescence, when the signs are already there that, when not recognised, will lead to a much more serious crisis in adulthood. I believe that the explosion of the psychotic crisis (with eventual hospitalisation) makes the therapeutic task much more difficult; it would be greatly facilitated if the analyst could intervene earlier.

The psychotic nucleus, in fact, acts on the rest of the personality like a cancerous metastasis that proliferates relentlessly. While it is

arduous and requires much time to gain access to the psychotic functioning, work on the delusional nucleus is unavoidable and, in particular, it is necessary to work with the patient through the outbreak of
the first crisis.

The patient's resistance to working on the past psychotic crisis can
be explained in various ways. Just as it is difficult for those who
survive a catastrophe to relive the terror and senselessness of the
violence suffered, so it is for the psychotic patient when he has to go
back in time and re-experience the catastrophic impact of his insane
thoughts. If the analyst wants to share the psychotic crisis with his
patient, he must be able to approach the area of suffering with the
utmost caution and sensitivity, since it can only be faced with enormous difficulty.

The patient's incapacity for remembering stems not only from the
pain of recognising himself as insane, but also from fear. Rethinking
the crisis means stimulating the same imagination that created the
delusion and that might once again invade him. He is not only afraid,
but also, when the psychotic crisis was experienced as an ecstatic illumination, perhaps attracted by its seductive qualities; the fascination
wielded by the psychotic nucleus explains the patient's acquiescence
to the delusion recurring.

Understanding the psychotic disorder has enlarged the horizons
and cognitive tools of psychoanalysis. With regard to this, it is sufficient to return to the notes, intuitions, and exclamations in Bion's *Cogitations* (1992), intent on capturing contemporaneously the essence of
the mathematician's and the psychotic's thinking. Bion's insight into
the alpha function and the beta elements, deriving from questions he
posed regarding the psychotic patient's incapacity to think, are useful
on a general theoretical level but remain applicable, in my humble
opinion, only in our work with this type of patient.

I believe that further understanding of the psychotic mind (and for
this I hope my colleagues will be increasingly engaged in the treatment of psychotics in an analytic setting) will produce not only an
advance in the analytic treatment in this sphere, but also a real epis-
temic opening up of the discipline itself. We are coming ever closer to
knowing how thought is formed and how emotions, which spring
from relations, are essential for the development of the intuitive skills
that are quite lacking in the psychotic mind.

CHAPTER SEVENTEEN

The therapeutic approach to the delusional experience

"An analyst wanting to treat psychotic patients needs additional training, and sometimes this may take several years. There are few analysts who find it easy to understand the psychotic patient"

(Rosenfeld, 1987, p. 59)

I consider delusion to be the result of a withdrawal from reality that began in childhood. This dissociated reality provides the necessary nourishment for the psychotic part of the personality, destined to take the upper hand during the course of the full-blown illness. In order to explore in greater depth the nature and dynamics of the delusional experience, I shall also explain why it is so very tenacious and why it tends to re-present itself even after the true psychotic episode has been overcome.

First, in this chapter, I describe the ways in which psychoanalytic theory has attempted to identify the nature of the delusional experience.

Theories of continuity and discontinuity

The various psychoanalytic conceptualisations about psychosis indicate an important distinction that calls for different therapeutic techniques.

As we know, contrasting standpoints regarding psychosis are represented within the psychoanalytic discipline by *continuity-based* and *discontinuity-based* theories (London, 1973): the first tend to consider psychotic behaviour as deriving from intrapsychic conflicts, similar in nature to those of the neurotic patient; discontinuous theories, instead, are *specific* because they infer a particular disorder.

According to the former theory, the delusion develops at the level of the unconscious functions that govern the patient's mental life (*the delusion as communication or expression of a conflict*) and can be considered a means by which the patient can communicate a hidden reality. This is how Freud (1911c) explains Schreber's illness as due to a childhood homosexual conflict that is manifested in the following sequences: intrapsychic conflict, anxiety, external projection, and regression to a state preceding fixation. Schreber's persecutory delusion would be nothing but a construction concealing his repressed homosexuality.

If the delusion is considered to be a communication, one must aim to decipher its implicit meaning, treating it, for example, as one treats dreams. Indeed, some authors have asked themselves whether the delusional construction preserves traces of childhood conflicts and is susceptible to being resolved by clarifying the nucleus of reality contained within it.

Following Freud's interpretative hypotheses, Niederland (1951) believes that Schreber was terrified of taking his father's position and felt increasingly helpless at the prospect of confronting him as a member of the Reichstag or as Senatspräsident.

The conviction that the delusion has communicative significance permeates the thinking of other authors, such as Israëls (1989), who believes that Paul Schreber's persecutory anxiety might be connected to the intrusive methods of his authoritarian father that return as hallucinations or delusions during his regression.

Discontinuity-based theories, on the other hand, postulate a clean divide between neurosis and psychosis, allowing the psychotic state to be conceived as a dissociated experience, which can be neither integrated nor transformed (*the delusion as construction of a dissociated reality*). The explosion of the mind, the real psychotic breakdown, would be nothing but the consequence of the same mechanism that supports the delusion.

From this point of view, the delusion is considered to be a dangerous parasitical construction that has to be investigated *as such* in order to contain and transform it, or to *deconstruct it*, as I propose to call it. In deconstructing the delusion, that is, reducing its power over the patient's mental functioning, we eliminate an obstacle to the resumption of the use of intuitive thought and of contact with emotional reality.

Freud (1924e) acknowledges that the delusion has a certain positive function; he postulates that when reality is obliterated through the id triumphing over the principle of reality, the ego must find something to replace it: the delusion would represent an attempt to reconstruct and reorganise reality.

One author who has moved away from the Freudian hypothesis of the delusion as an attempt at reconstruction is Federn (1952); he claims that the delusion *does not correspond to an attempt at reconstruction*, but is the consequence of the falsification of psychic reality. Federn maintains that, in psychosis, the main damage lies in the loss of the investment of the ego's boundaries, with the consequent invasion of hallucinated reality.

For this reason, Federn suggests that our therapeutic work with psychotic patients should not entail *interpretations of meaning*, including transferral ones (for him, therefore, the delusion is not communication), because these increase the confusion of an ego already too dispersed. Instead, our work should aim at strengthening the patient's sense of identity, protecting him from excessive anxiety and improving his capacity to think. Regarding free associations, since the psychotic patient is besieged by an excess of sense and meaning, these should not be encouraged but limited. One of Federn's most important propositions is that "in neurosis we want to eliminate repression, in psychosis we want to restore it" (1952, p. 136). It is not a matter of "making the unconscious conscious, but [of] making the unconscious again" (Federn, 1952, p. 178). In other words, Federn postulates that you cannot interpret the delusion because the psychotic patient has lost the capacity to symbolise; instead, it is necessary to contain his tendency to let himself be seduced by an excess of meaning.

The psychotic and non-psychotic part of the personality

Freud (1940a) was the first to describe the functioning of two parts of the personality in psychosis:

> Two psychical attitudes have been formed instead of a single one – one, the normal one, which takes account of reality, and another, which under the influence of the instincts detaches the ego from reality. The two exist alongside of each other. The issue depends on their relative strength. (p. 202)

We have authors such as Katan and Bion to thank for further exploring the dynamics of psychotic and normal functioning.

Katan (1954) has studied in particular the pre-psychotic phase of the illness, when a part of the personality is still able to remain in contact with reality. The author states,

> . . . the delusion does not possess an unconscious . . . One may distinguish between a neurotic and a delusional projection. The neurotic projection serves the purpose of warding off the id . . . The delusional form of projection has a wholly different structure. . . . To put it differently, although not entirely correctly: part of the id has become outer world. The delusion is a sign that in the pre-psychotic phase or in the non-psychotic layer contact has been broken off, and the formation of the delusion is the result of the attempt to repair the break with reality. (p. 126)

As I have already mentioned, Bion (1957), too, distinguishes between the psychotic and the non-psychotic personality and, in particular, outlines the differences in their functioning. The neurotic part functions by assimilation, introjection, and discrimination, while the psychotic part proceeds by violent projections that aim to get rid of the accumulation of psychic elements that it cannot "digest".

Linking up with Klein's intuitions (1930) regarding the incapacity to symbolise and with Segal (1956) regarding the impossibility of the psychotic facing up to the depressive position, Bion asserts that being unable to tolerate pain pushes the patient to destroy the function of thought. While the neurotic patient uses repression to relegate the negative experience to the unconscious, the psychotic patient destroys the tools that would allow the unconscious to understand the psychic experiences. According to Bion, in fact, the main function of the unconscious is to transform sensory data into symbolic elements; if sensory data are not transformed, psychic life would be impossible.

The psychotic patient cannot unconsciously repress and work through the data of the experience (he cannot *dream*) and, consequently, he cannot derive any benefit from it. It is interesting to note that other authors, for example Abraham and Federn, while starting from different standpoints, reach similar conclusions about the failed function of repression.

For this reason, the apparent accessibility for the observer to what could be considered an open manifestation of the psychotic unconscious (an unconscious without repression) is, I contrast, the result of the failed transformation of sensory data. Due to the destruction of the alpha function, the psychotic patient is in a state of serious psychic deficiency.

At this point, the distinction between unaware and unconscious is essential. Here, I will make a difference between consciousness and awareness, two concepts that are held to be comparable.[19]

While in normal conditions unconscious and unaware coincide (we are unaware, that is, we do not know our unconscious thoughts), in psychosis the patient is conscious (that is, he perceives his delusion and fixes it in his memory), but he is not aware of its meaning. This leads to my belief that our analytic work with psychotic patients must attempt to make them develop an *awareness* (and not a *consciousness*) that they have lacked since infancy.

Persecutory anxiety

I now turn to the problem of the specific nature of the delusion and the singular way in which it is constructed, commenting on a brief clinical fragment from the analysis of a patient.

* * *

Now thirty-seven years old, Giovanni began analysis at four sessions a week six years ago, after a period of hospitalisation for a psychotic episode.

At the beginning he was completely delusional and interpretative, immersed in a persecutory perception of reality. This extremely strong interpretative tendency reached the point of contaminating, at times, even the analytic relationship, with the risk of a psychotic transference that could have made it impossible to continue the analysis.

The persecutory delusional episode, which had begun before treatment, had appeared after a period of megalomania in which Giovanni had believed he could become powerful and famous, destined to dominate the world. After disagreeing with a colleague, he had felt persecuted by the organisation of his rival, who controlled him with hidden microphones and video cameras and was plotting all possible ways of killing him (poison in his glass at the bar, toxic gas at home, lethal radiations from his computer, and so on).

*   *   *

I would now like to relate a recent sequence to demonstrate exactly how tenacious the delusional experience can be.

*   *   *

Giovanni is much better now and not only from a symptomatic point of view. He has come out of the threatening dominion of the psychotic state and, with the help of analytic work, has begun to construct his personal identity and to understand, at least in part, his emotional world.

Naturally, this process is by no means linear. The delusion still presents itself in a transitory way; it changes its contents and its representations according to the events in his life but—an important element—it is constantly brought to analysis to be worked through. This allows both Giovanni and myself to put the delusion at a safe distance and to evade its power. The delusional experience is still a second reality for Giovanni, although not as threatening as in his first years of analysis; it is a reality that he enters but that he can easily come out of.

I said that this patient was much improved; in analysis he maintains good dependence and communicates with me. He has succeeded in making significant stable bonds with his peers and has recently had an important encounter with a young woman: a few weeks ago, he decided to buy a bigger bed so they could sleep together. So, he went to a shop and the assistant showed him a number of mattresses, among which he indicated one that seemed the most suitable. At this point, Giovanni felt alarmed and felt himself plunging into the delusional experience.

*   *   *

I try to understand what has reawakened the persecutory terror. To an external observer, it is difficult to understand the connection between the suggestion of a mattress and the emergence of the persecution and the patient himself would have found it difficult to provide any useful clues if he had been asked.

For me, seeing that I have listened to Giovanni for a long time now and clearly have in mind the delusional experiences that emerged before and during his analysis, a mattress and a bed immediately seemed very significant, not for their symbolic value, but precisely because they were such concrete visual images. I immediately connected the patient's anxiety to one, among the many, of his past delusional perceptions; I see him again, way back, unable to sleep, tormented by persecution and hallucinatory perceptions. At night, he was terrified of the evil power of his persecutors: he was sure that a certain luminescence emanating from the *mattress* was due to the presence of a radioactive material placed in his *bed* by his enemies to kill him. By indicating a mattress to buy, the shop assistant, therefore, was trying to repeat the persecution; he was potentially an emissary of whoever wants the patient's death.

An important and systematic part of the analytic work involves the patient's propensity to succumb to the terror or seduction of the delusion, so it is very important to work constantly on reconstructing the first psychotic episode that leads to the patient's readiness to be delusional.

This aspect of therapy must not be neglected for any reason at all and it is necessary to proceed with it in the most systematic way possible. In my opinion, I believe it is essential for the patient to face up to this task so that he can gradually learn how to defend himself and establish a distance from the psychotic functioning.

In general, when the psychotic episode has exhausted itself, the patient tends to preserve the precarious balance achieved, even if this involves numerous limitations; he learns to hold himself aloof from those emotional experiences that could destabilise him and senses that there is a boundary beyond which he cannot push himself. For this reason, he keeps relationships and affective investments that could trigger new psychotic outbursts well under control and knows that, if he ventures beyond his own Pillars of Hercules, it would be catastrophic. A relapse into psychosis is fostered precisely by progress that the psychic structure cannot tolerate.

I have included this clinical example to demonstrate the tenacity of the delusional experience and to show how it will return and threaten the patient yet again. Freud (1940a), too, points out that the delusion is always latent but tenaciously preserves its power:

> If the relation is reversed [or if the part in contact with reality prevails] then there is an apparent cure of the delusional disorder. Actually it has only retreated into the unconscious – just as numerous observations lead us to believe that the delusion existed ready-made for a long time before its manifest irruption. (p. 202)

Reflecting on this short passage serves the making of some observations on the structuring of the delusion and its reappearance.

In the case of this patient, Giovanni, the mnemonic trigger that fuels his delusion does not correspond to a memory inserted in a context; it seems to be a foreign body, a radioactive fragment capable of still contaminating his world. Despite the years of analysis and reflection on his capacity to alter reality (both in a grandiose and a persecutory sense) the delusional splinter is still parked in his mind and persists as a dangerous source of madness.

In the fragment above, the delusion was quickly re-formed on the basis of elementary associative connections. The word *mattress* evoked the delusional scene of the past and brought the persecutory sequence sharply into focus. Note how the *word* has here become a concrete fact. The mattress is not one among many, but that particular mattress on which the patient believes he risked dying. Words, here, resemble stones or, as Freud would say, *representation of the thing* replaces *representation of the word*. Starting from this differentiation, Freud (1915e) suggests that in the schizophrenic disorder *words* enter into the so-called primary process. Having disinvested both the representation of the thing and of the word, in seeking to recover, schizophrenics take "a path that leads to the object *via* the verbal part of it, but then find themselves obliged to be content with words instead of things" (p. 204). In exactly the same way, the psychotic treats words, which are condensed and replaced, as though they were things. In my opinion, Freud's intuitions on this point are invaluable for understanding how words and verbal associations are capable of concretely reinforcing the delusional image. Similarly, in the past in the case of Giovanni, merely the word *oil*, casually pronounced by someone he was talking

to, triggered the same delusional state of mind (his presumed persecutors were Iranian, a country rich in oil).

The delusion is undoubtedly sparked not by a thought, but by a
vision, a sensory experience, a sequence of terrifying visual images,
which have been indelibly impressed, that return to centre stage and
flood the psyche. To repeat Giovanni's words once more, "This insight
springs from your very innards and floods your mind." During the
delusional experience, the patient, in fact, does not think; he *sees* or
hears: the sensory images replace the perception of psychic reality. The
self dissolves and, with it, the capacity to think.

As I hope to have shown, the delusion, with all its many facets,
remains in the psyche as something terrible that happened and is
destined *not to be worked through* because it is dominated by traumatic
anxiety.

The difference between dream and delusion

Despite their apparent similarity, a delusion is the opposite of a
dream. The dreams of psychotic patients, when they appear, cannot
be considered as dreams because they are not the result of a process
of symbolisation and there is no inner mental space to contain them;
they often incorporate psychotic material and, at times, allow us to
glimpse a delusion in the making, as I attempt to illustrate below.

Money-Kyrle (1971) claims that a tendency to transform reality is
inherent in the human psyche; psychoanalysis should aim to help the
patient overcome the obstacles that conceal what is innately known.
As a result, a region of the psyche would preserve the unconscious
perception of truth intact, despite the defensive distortion.

Yet, however efficiently Money-Kyrle's concept of psychic functioning delineates the dynamics of the repression of psychic truth in
normal and neurotic individuals, it is not suitable for the psychotic
situation. While his claim that illness derives from an unconscious
delusion is true, it is also true that a distinction must be made between
the various levels of the distortion of reality: the *conscious*, the *unconscious*, and the truly *delusional*.

During the course of regular analytic therapies, it is possible to see
that, while the analysand gradually succeeds in perceiving his own
psychic reality and in developing the capacity to understand his

emotional truth, some of his beliefs are revealed to be false. This is the growing experience that allows the personality to be integrated and enriched.

In my opinion, though, this path is not possible for psychotic patients because their psychotic constructions do not refer back to split or repressed omnipotent fantasies that can be reintegrated.

There is no continuity between the unconscious thought, which helps to perceive psychic reality, and the delusional activity. They are two opposing functions.

Like delusions, *pathological constructions* tend to distort the perception of psychic reality to the point of destroying it by constructing a rival perceptive world; their aim is to create a neo-reality that appears to be better and more desirable, which is why their colonising action is not evident to the patient, who, instead, is passively attracted to it.

Delusions are difficult to demolish because they are sensory constructions rather than thought generated. The patient is convinced they are real because the delusional and hallucinatory construction derives its semblance of reality from the mind's self-arousing and sensory activity. In fact, in the psychotic state, the mind is not used as a tool for thought but as a sensory organ. Since delusions and hallucinations have the same quality as ordinary perceptions produced by stimulation of the perceptive organs by external objects, they present themselves to the patient as *reality* even though they are not *real* for the external observer because they are not shared.

The nature of the delusion

The delusion is intrinsically a psychopathological construction, a *mental state* that cannot be treated by interpretative work directed at illustrating its hidden meaning. Both external and internal reality are altered in the delusion and, thus, also the sense of personal identity. We could say that the delusion is a falsification the patient is unaware of that imposes itself on consciousness, causing a progressive alteration of the sense of reality.

The delusion must be deconstructed, not interpreted, because it is a neo-construction that cannot be symbolised or integrated. It is situated outside the "dreaming function of wakefulness" that allows us to carry out emotional transformations that contribute to integrating our sense of identity and perception of being. The delusion derives from the mind being conquered by the dissociated reality, "the other reality", into which the patient has fled a long time ago.

Badaracco (1983), who has devoted part of his professional life to treating psychosis, expresses similar ideas when he writes,

> Clinical experience has led us to believe that the intermediate links are in effect lacking, as if the process of therapeutic working through were in fact one of dismantling the psychotic productions so that the components can subsequently be recomposed in a different form by means of the therapeutic process itself. (p. 700)

Likewise, I also propose working by means of deconstructing or demolishing. Deconstruction (a term symmetrical to psychopathological construction) allows us to study in detail and to recognise step by step how the psychopathological construction was built up and develops by accurately examining also the present and past emotional states preparatory to the delusion.

Demolishing the force of the delusion is accompanied by the acquisition of functions of awareness, which gradually allow the patient to "see" and, therefore, to evade, the lure of the psychopathological construction. Maintaining this capacity over time, apart from constant shifts in perspective, guarantees that the delusional experience, if it reappears, is recognised and made transformable. For this type of analytic work, intrapsychic analytic interpretations are invaluable; they do not call for symbolic meanings or concern the transference, but continually describe to the patient the dynamics of the conquest of his mind by the psychotic organisation.

It is not true, as is often said, that the delusion manifests itself as an intuition that presents itself with blinding clarity and for this reason is immediately accepted by the patient. It is not like this. The delusion does not spring forth like Minerva from Jove's head, but is prepared by a series of connected associations.

Initially, these signs are not taken seriously; they are ignored or, in other words, split from awareness. They only become visible in a later moment when they present themselves in an apparently coherent sequence. When a certain critical point has been reached, the microtransformations "suddenly" converge into the delusional illuminating flash.

A clear case of dissociating judgement with an aim of preserving the delusion can be found in the memoirs of President Schreber (1955). Although able to comprehend other patients' mental states, he has no understanding of his own. He writes,

> I am fully aware that other people may be tempted to think that I am pathologically conceited; I know very well that this very tendency to relate everything to oneself, to bring everything that happens into connection with one's person, is a common phenomenon among mental patients . . . But in my case the very reverse obtains. Since God entered into nerve-contact with me exclusively, I became in a way for God the only human being, or simply the human being around whom everything turns, to whom everything that happens must be related and who therefore, from his point of view, must also relate all things to himself. (p. 187)

Manipulation of the organs of consciousness

Psychosis and withdrawal into a pleasurable state are synonymous, in my opinion. If the attraction towards the psychosis was not initially pleasurable, we would not be able to understand the readiness to become psychotic.

As Freud has stated and as Bion has reminded us, we possess an *organ of consciousness* that is capable of understanding psychic reality; within certain limits we can manipulate and alter this organ, similar to that which happens in all defensive procedures. In fact, we can say that the psychotic patient does not use his mind to think, but to produce sensations. In this way, hallucinations are produced, which are at first pleasurable but then become a source of anxiety: the patient "sees" with the eyes of his mind; he "hears" with the ears of his mind.

Manipulation of the organs of psychic perception reaches extreme levels, to the extent of creating special worlds in which the patient is ensnared: for example, states of sexualised well-being, of perverse pleasure, or of delusional reality. The withdrawal, however, is never idyllic for very long; an initial exhilarating phase is followed by a terrifying plunge into anxiety.

The alteration to the organ of consciousness produced by the psychotic defence turns out to be catastrophic; indeed, to maintain the omnipotence and persevere in his flight from reality, the patient must increasingly violate his perceptive organs, finishing by destroying them and being left defenceless. This is what happens in the psychotic state.

Difficulty in working through

Why is the delusional experience so very tenacious that it can resist being worked through? I shall now linger, for a moment only, on the grandiose delusion of persecution, since, for other delusional forms, the matter might well be different.

I believe that the mental apparatus is destructured, at times permanently, when it experiences the level of terror reached during the delusional process. This is why the delusion is tantamount to an emotional trauma destined to damage the mental apparatus and to perpetuate anxiety. Delusional memory is extraordinarily similar to traumatic memory.

Van der Kolk (1994; Van der Kolk et al., 1996) suggests that traumatic memories constitute indelible sensory images, bodily sensations, sounds, and olfactory and visual impressions separated from the rest of the psyche. They are dissociated from consciousness but can unexpectedly burst forth when the traumatic memory is activated, emerging from their state of encapsulation.

Memories and feelings linked to traumatic experiences are, therefore, radically separated (dissociated) from the rest of the psyche because they are unbearable. The result is that the dissociative defence, by inhibiting perception of what has happened, prevents the process of working through the trauma, and, in fact, perpetuates it.

This also occurs in psychosis, which, for me, is tantamount to an endo-traumatic fact. The patient "recovers" from the psychotic crisis, but recovers *defectively*; the psychotic episode is dissociated (also thanks to the action of psychotropic drugs) and remains, not worked through, ready to re-emerge.

In the case of the patient Giovanni, even in quite an advanced stage of analysis (the fourth year), the traumatic anxiety quickly re-emerged thanks to associative connections of contiguity, assonance, and resemblance.

The words ("mattress", "oil") became concrete stimuli that, thanks to their associative semantic aura (similarity, contiguity, temporal or spatial links), reactivated the psychotic anxiety that had remained fixed without being able to be worked through.

I have already said that the patient is easily colonised by the delusion and that this fact poses specific problems to those dealing with the therapy of psychosis. A part of the mind exists that is virtually inaccessible to the analyst, in which the patient continues to build up his psychosis; this is why I emphasise the importance of the communication of psychotic dreams (Capozzi & De Masi, 2001), because these often describe quite clearly, with no attempt at camouflage, the withdrawal and colonising action of the psychotic part.

Two clinical fragments

I now present a brief fragment from a male patient's case and the more detailed clinical case of a female patient. Both have had psychotic episodes that they are trying to recover from with the help of analysis, although they still feel attracted to them. In both cases, the dream is like a shop window that displays the content of the delusion linked to arousing sensations suggested by the psychotic part together with anxious feelings that derive from the healthy part.

*   *   *

The first case is that of a young man aged twenty-six, who had a delusional episode in which he felt "enlightened".[20] The Pope had let Gianni know that he had invented the "morkema", a language enabling deaf-mutes to communicate among themselves and with the world at large. But, some time later, this flash of illumination turned into persecution: perhaps he was not really a genius; perhaps the devil had laid a trap so that he would die. Gianni said that a "voice" suggested to him that he should kill himself because he would certainly carry out an extraordinary deed, but only after his death.

After some months of analytic work on his delusional ideation, Gianni seemed to be less anxious and began to recognise how an urge for grandiose exaltation had turned into the persecutory fear of becoming a devil responsible for having destroyed order in the universe.

This is the dream:

"I woke up, full of anxiety. I dreamt that I had a huge belly because I was pregnant and then I had a second belly that moved like a book, with another baby. The feeling of the dream was very pleasurable."

*   *   *

In this dream, Gianni describes the psychotic part taking hold of the healthy part. The patient says that, despite the exhilarating state that characterised the dream, he was full of anxiety on waking. Using the *opposing emotions of the dream and of waking* (pleasure and anxiety), the analyst can show the patient how, when he lets himself be seduced by the alluring enticements of the delusional omnipotence, the perceptive healthy part of the self is immediately alarmed and anxious.

Pleasure in the delusion

I now comment on a clinical case, observed in supervision, in which it is relatively easy to identify some characteristics of the psychotic state and of its cunning in ensnaring the patient who, in his turn, is ready to deceive the analyst.

*   *   *

Some months before the start of analysis, Agnese had been admitted to the psychiatric department of the hospital in her town for an acute psychotic episode. The apparent symptoms were characterised by auditory and visual hallucinations and by an ideational disorder of a delusional nature that inclined strongly to interpretation and magic thoughts. The medical history gleaned from her relatives when she was admitted was not very extensive. She remained only a short time in the ward and, when she was discharged, she seemed to have recovered a sufficient hold on reality, although she still appeared very evanescent.

The psychotic episode manifested itself suddenly and Agnese rapidly demonstrated an apparent recovery. She was entrusted as an outpatient to a psychiatrist who prescribed psychotropic drugs and sent her to a female analyst some months later for therapy. After about two months of face-to-face consultations, Agnese accepted the proposal to start analysis at four sessions a week, lying on a couch. The analyst believed it was also useful to talk to her parents to inform them of the difficulties inherent to the therapy and to sound out their willingness to support their daughter. The mother, in particular, appeared very anxious and during therapy it became clear that she tended to blame Agnese for her admission to hospital and for her illness.

At the beginning, Agnese never missed a session. In the first months, she was accompanied by her mother, then, gradually, she managed to come alone. Initially, she seems inexpressive and fearful, perhaps still immersed in a delusional atmosphere that she tends to conceal. She is sad and lifeless as though, on coming out of the psychotic crisis, she has become depressed, empty, and without direction. In some sessions, she lets a few memories of the difficult relationship with her parents emerge. She says that when she was fourteen she had been hit by her mother and forcefully taken back home because she had been surprised holding hands and kissing a boy from her school whom she had fallen for. Agnese says that since then she has always avoided going out with a boy because she is frightened of the possible reaction of her parents.

In fact, during adolescence she never attempted to achieve an autonomous life apart from her parents. She has never been on holiday alone or with a group of friends. Moreover, she rarely went out with her girlfriends and this made her feel even more isolated from the world.

We can suppose that it was then that Agnese began to construct her psychic withdrawal, which took on the semblance of a love nest in which to take shelter, a fantastic world in which symbols and signs reinforced what she herself was creating. The delusion that led to her admission to hospital was, in fact, of an erotic nature. The protagonist was an old school friend who had fallen in love with her, followed her, spoke to her, was present everywhere, but who was never visible because, in her words, he always hid himself from her eyes. Agnese's mental state was characterised by frenzy stimulated by visual and auditory hallucinations that referred to the presence and to the signs left by her loved one.

Marco, the protagonist of the delusion, had indeed been one of her schoolmates. But the striking aspect is that Agnese remembers that he was the leader of an aggressive gang that constantly made fun of her and helped to isolate her even more in class. Agnese's delusional withdrawal helped her to completely overturn the frustrating reality she had experienced: Marco now loves her and cannot live without her.

* * *

I now describe the material of a session from the fourth month of analysis.

> The patient enters, smiling and rather evanescent: "I will describe my dream: I was living inside a video game; the walls opened and closed at my commands depending on whether I said 'open file, close file'. But when I opened it, some people approached wanting to come in; they were dangerous. It was a constant opening and closing. I wanted to open so that I could get out but I was obliged to close to protect myself. I am always afraid. Even yesterday when I went to Milan with my mother I was afraid, and when I got home I breathed a sigh of relief."

It would seem that, in this dream, Agnese is describing her psychotic functioning: she can create a video game that replaces psychic reality, opening it and closing it at will. But then the psychotic system becomes threatening: Agnese can no longer master it and risks being held prisoner with no way of escape.

In a subsequent session, about a month before the summer holidays:

> "I'm happy today because I had a nice dream, not an anxious one. I was with my friends from high school, but only those I liked, including Diana and Luciana. We were at a school near the sea. I had to do a computer test; my friends had a maths test. At a certain point I confess to them what had happened in September. Then I ask them to get the medicine that I have to take. They are very kind to me, they understand me, but the absurd thing about the dream is that Marco arrives too [the character from the delusion], and he doesn't make fun of me or treat me badly; in fact he tells me that he would like to go out with me as long as I stop giving myself airs. Then I woke up calm and peaceful."

The dream is, apparently, calm and positive. In the first part, Agnese manages to talk to her friends about her psychotic crisis and even remembers the antipsychotic medicine she has to take. But, at this point, Marco, the protagonist of her amorous delusion, unexpectedly appears.

It really does seem to be a peaceful dream, but closer attention reveals it to be decidedly ambiguous. Why does Marco appear unexpectedly in the dream? Why is the school at the seaside?

In the face of this material the question the analyst must ask himself is whether the patient is not trying to convince her interlocutor (as she does with her two friends in the dream) that everything is going well, that she has recovered her peace of mind, while in actual fact she is secretly preparing another delusional meeting with Marco on the brink of the summer holidays.

In the next session, Agnese seems apparently quite calm:

> "It's a period in which I'm thinking about the future; two simple things make me euphoric. I'll give you an example: I bought a cream for cellulite to use in the summer and it's a fixed thought, I do nothing but think about the holidays. I bought a new swimsuit. I spend many hours in front of the mirror. It's such an exhilarating thought, it makes me feel hyperactive. Then I started chatting to Daniele, and we spoke about everything, films, theatre, sport."

> The analyst comments that in fact the patient's thoughts are pleasurable at the beginning and then they become morbid and bad.

> Agnese replies, "I can send them away only if I take a bit of a sedative. Every time I go to the seaside I always dream of meeting someone who will overturn my life and who I can perhaps run away with . . ."

The conclusion we can draw from this sequence of sessions is that the patient is preparing another psychotic episode, since the summer break is approaching and her analyst will not be there. The cellulite cream might allude to the beginning of a new euphoric sexual phase.

In fact, in a very short time, the same delusional atmosphere of the first psychotic episode is recreated. Agnese begins to miss sessions and, while she tells her parents she is going to the analyst, prefers to wander about town in a para-delusional way. Only a prompt and attentive psychiatric intervention and the resumption of regular sessions, after only a short holiday break, will prevent re-admission to hospital.

This brief clinical example serves to demonstrate how the delusion, once established, tends to re-present itself.

In this case, the lure of the aroused and ecstatic state was strongly enticing and the approaching summer break from analysis reinforced the psychotic part. Agnese has always lived a spare and isolated life and so seems to perceive the delusional part as an intoxicating experience of freedom.

In the very moment in which she produces the dream of the school at the seaside, the patient is at risk; the delusional part has already created a collusive complicity with the healthy part. In parallel to the patient's reticence, which is not a good sign (indeed, it often constitutes the determining element of a new relapse), the dream in this case reveals the machinations of the psychotic part.

So, the analyst's skill in successfully grasping traces of the psychotic transformation in the dream is absolutely crucial.

This clinical material about Agnese exemplifies how the dreams of some patients can acquire the predictive value of an impending psychotic crisis. Investigation into, and working through, how the delusion forms itself should be one of the essential points in Agnese's analysis, too. This work must be done constantly and for a long period of time.

The importance of the psychotic dream

In this sense, as I have attempted to demonstrate in the brief clinical fragments, psychotic dreams are very useful because they constitute the *real communication to the analyst* that is not otherwise possible while the patient is an accomplice of, and subject to, the delusional organisation. From this viewpoint, *while the delusion conceals, the dream communicates.*

The meaning of a psychotic dream, which does not refer to the search for a symbolic content, but to the creation of the psychotic state, can convey a communication that proves indispensable for working on the psychotic nucleus and on the patient's propensity to be delusional.

The representation of the psychosis contained in the "dream" and the way in which the patient lets himself be enticed by it can be worked on at length and at subsequent moments.

To conclude, if the delusion is a psychopathological construction aimed at transforming psychic reality, the psychotic "dream", which also represents the pressure of the delusion that can colonise the ego, can become, for the patient, one of the tools he has available for *communicating* what is happening and for being helped out of the seductive clutches of the psychosis. So, the dream, and not the delusion, represents the means for communicating and for beginning to understand what operations and ways the patient has for entering into a psychotic state.

CHAPTER EIGHTEEN

The problematic position of the transference in the psychotic state

"Delusional production positions itself in a space that is neither the inner space of the psyche, nor external space, and not even intermediate or transitional space . . ."

(Racamier, 2000, p. 873)

The psychotic transference results from a pre-existing delusion that invades the analytic setting and relationship: the analyst becomes an object of the delusion and his interpretative function vanishes. The psychotic part that has overcome the rest of the personality destroys the patient's intuitive and self-observation capacities and obstructs the analytic work.

This chapter discusses the onset of psychotic episodes during analysis and, in particular, the delusional transference which, once established, tends to bring the analytic process to a dangerous impasse.

This subject is not widely discussed in contemporary psychoanalytic literature, and neither do many recent papers deal with the analytic therapy of psychotic patients.

Past contributions

In earlier psychoanalytic literature, the onset of a psychotic state during therapy was often the object of close examination and produced many differing contributions.

In 1965, a Panel of the American Psychoanalytic Society was held in New York with the theme "Severe regressive states during analysis" under the presidency of Frosch (Weinshel, 1966).

The main objective of this conference was to understand whether the regressive disorganisation manifested in serious cases, however turbulent and difficult to manage, could be considered a necessary stage towards the patient's improvement or a dangerous occurrence to be expunged as quickly as possible.

Opinions on this point varied enormously: some participants claimed that the serious regressions that burst forth during analysis are of no help to the patient at all; others, in contrast, believed that the regressive experience in seriously ill patients should be considered an inevitable preliminary act for reintegration to upper levels of adaptation.

Another issue that emerged from the Panel was whether it was possible to intuit this type of development from the patient's history and from the initial consultations, or whether it was destined to be discovered only during treatment.

Other issues raised questioned what other events might facilitate or determine these risky reactions and what the relationship is between this condition, the real transference, and the so-called transference psychosis.

On re-reading the papers presented in this important Panel, it is clear that, while the times were not yet ripe for reaping useful clinical answers, the fundamental questions were posed in an extremely clear and explicit way. These issues are still valid for us today.

The model

As mentioned in the previous chapter, my model for understanding the evolution of the delusion and, consequently, the psychotic transference is based on the contrast that Bion (1957) drew our attention to between the healthy and the psychotic parts of the personality. In the case of psychosis, the psychotic part not only dominates the healthy part, but progressively colonises and engulfs it until it disappears. The psychotic withdrawal is not always obvious to the surrounding context. The child destined to become psychotic can seem calm, although certainly isolated and not very communicative, and so his parents generally ignore the fact that he is living in a psychic retreat (Steiner, 1993), in a reality of dissociated fantasy. As Resnik (2001) points out, the psychotic patient lives in constant oscillation between two worlds: the real one and another one that resembles an uninterrupted dream.

The meaning of the crisis

Instead, from a different standpoint from the one I have just illustrated, some authors believe that the regression manifested during the psychotic crisis is a positive occurrence, almost an integral part of the analytic process.

In 1958, Little authored a paper on the transference psychosis, or the "delusional transference", which manifests itself in people with character disorders, perversions, psychosomatic illnesses, mental disorders, the borderlines, and so on. The delusional transference does not have the "as if" characteristic of the neurotic transference and lacks capacity for symbolising; consequently, transference interpretations in this state are ineffective. Little goes on to say that dream analysis, too, is counterproductive, because it deals with dreams that contain only defence mechanisms and whose manifest content leads to numerous associations but not to the latent content. In dreams of this type, the manifest content and the latent content are one and the same thing, so that the manifest content corresponds to the dream-thought. Despite these characteristics that render the therapy highly complex, Little is convinced that the patient must regress to a state of non-integration, of non-differentiation between the self and the object, between mind and body.

Searles (1963), too, believes that regression and symbiosis are necessary for resuming ego development, and intends regression as a return to a preceding state of the ego, or to a previous psychosis, or to a previous fixation point.

When writing of the transference psychosis, Searles intends the development of a psychotic episode during the therapy of an apparently healthy person whose ego structure is of a borderline type. The transference psychosis distorts the relationship between patient and therapist and prevents them relating to each other as two distinct beings.

Other authors, however, criticise the concept that sees in regression a significant phase of therapy and think that this event represents a negative fact that must be arrested as rapidly as possible. It is not easy, however, to distinguish therapeutic regressions from pathological ones.

In 1966, Gustav Bychowski postulates that the transference psychosis, which should in any case always be considered a therapeutic failure, is characterised by the completely delusional psychotic distortions projected on to the figure of the analyst: in the neurotic transference the patient knows it is a fantasy, whereas, in the psychotic transference, he believes it to be reality. The author claims that a psychotic nucleus corresponding to a primitive archaic ego—full of narcissism and grandiosity, and also of non-neutralised aggression and destructive hostility—lies at the basis of the psychotic transference. This archaic ego would be the result of regressive processes that the ego submitted itself to as a defence against early traumas.

In his article "Reconstruction and mastery in the transference psychosis", Wallerstein (1967) states that the transference psychosis is an expression of the problems that arise when borderline or clearly psychotic patients are analysed; the analyst is frequently included in the delusion in this type of transference. The author describes with great precision two of his cases, two women with a neurotic pathology (one hysterical, the other seriously obsessive), judged suitable for classic analysis, who had developed a delusional transference. Both had lost their fathers in childhood in traumatic ways that had not been worked through due to the family context's incapacity. In both cases, the transference psychosis signalled the return of the original trauma, and the psychotic regression had a reconstructive function.

Psychotic transference and transference psychosis

In distinguishing the *psychotic transference* from the *transference psychosis*, Kernberg (1975) and Rosenfeld (1979) made important progress regarding both the problem of psychotic manifestations during therapy and the relationship between the transference and psychosis.

The psychotic transference involves the inclusion of the figure of the analyst in the patient's delusional world. The transference psychosis, instead, is a *psychosis* that is limited only to the *transference*: in this state, the patient develops delusional ideas, psychotic behaviour, or hallucinations only within the analytic situation; the loss of being able to distinguish reality does not interfere too greatly with his life, which remains apparently unchanged.

The patient develops aggressiveness and hate only for the analyst who, experienced as a source of anxiety and terror, is feared and attacked in delusional ways. Interpretations are misunderstood to such a degree that communication is quite impossible; the analyst feels impotent and overwhelmed by the violent development of the psychotic process that he is dragged into.

However, Kernberg and Rosenfeld regard the transference psychosis in two different ways.

Kernberg thinks that it is an inevitable development of the analytic relationship with a borderline patient, who repeats the unconscious pathogenic relationships of his past; his confusion stems from the ego lacking boundaries, typical of these conditions. This is why the transference psychosis has to be halted, establishing rules and limitations for the patient's aggressive expressions.

Rosenfeld, instead, advances the hypothesis that traumatised borderline patients present a very sadistic superego. When this superego is projected into the analyst, the transference psychosis develops: gripped by terrible anxiety, the patient hears the analyst telling him that he (patient) is totally bad. His anxiety has to do with his fear of disintegrating, of dying, of going completely mad, or of being made mad by the analyst. Rosenfeld postulates that the transference psychosis manifests itself in traumatised borderline patients thanks to an ill-timed interpretation of the destructive aspects; these patients develop a persecutory delusion because the analyst actually behaved, even though unknowingly, as a destructive superego.

In brief, we can assume that the transference psychosis develops in borderline patients when the analyst repeatedly does not understand the patient, who then feels attacked as though the analyst's mistake was intentional, made expressly to injure him or make him go mad. Most probably, the trauma the patient experiences in the analytic relationship repeats a similar condition suffered in childhood.

The psychotic transference, on the other hand, develops not through any iatrogenic facilitation, but because a pre-existing delusion progresses to invade the analytic space as well.

Delimitations of the boundaries

Here, I would like to point out that I am writing specifically about the delusional transference; this does not mean that the non-psychotic transference and the corresponding countertransference are not also present in some stages, and they have to be treated in the customary way. In other words, we are dealing with two realities—the psychotic one and the non-psychotic one—that exist side by side.

Some analysts describe a countertransference that, in the therapy of psychotic patients, takes on the characteristics of an overwhelming experience: a state of confusion in which the boundaries of the self and the sense of identity are precarious (Lombardi, 2005). Lombardi (2003) vividly describes his countertransference stemming from one of his psychotic patients' violent projections that made him feel such acute vertigo and nausea that he had to clutch on to the arms of his chair to stop himself feeling projected into space. Resnik (2001), too, points out that during the psychosis, the bodily image disintegrates and the patient loses his feeling of being a person; all this is recorded in the countertransference that thus becomes, for the analyst, a compass capable of monitoring the direction in which the patient is moving.

The delusional transference

I have previously stated that the psychotic patient remains anchored to a sensory reality that is difficult to transform into thought, which corresponds to an incapacity to dream.

As I will attempt to show further on, this deficit prevents the psychotic from producing a transference endowed with emotional and symbolical value, an understanding of which can be given back to him via interpretation.

The psychotic transference involves the inclusion of the figure of the analyst into the patient's delusional world. Up to a certain moment, the patient is able to distinguish the delusional state from the transference, but then this faculty diminishes; in other words, the pre-existing delusion develops and expands to incorporate the analyst. During the psychotic state, the analyst can become a threatening character (as in a persecutory transference) or appear as a seductive person who lures or arouses the patient (as in a delusional erotic transference). The danger of this situation lies in the fact that the analyst loses his state of being a person distinct from the patient and is divested of his analytic function. To win it back, he has to get out of the position he has been confined in by the patient. Even if, as I have said, the appearance of a psychotic transference is always a hazardous occurrence, it is necessary to work on it in order to understand how the patient constructed it.

* * *

Giovanni[21] went through a psychotic episode of a delusional nature that manifested itself when he was abroad and whose symptoms became partially dormant following pharmacological treatment. The persecutory delusion, which appeared after a phase of megalomaniac expansion, was triggered by an argument with a foreign colleague who became the leader of a band of conspirators who wanted to kill him.

Although recovered to a certain extent and having taken up part-time consultancy work (for which he leaves home every day and meets people), Giovanni functions as though he is suspended between two adjacent psychic realities, one of which can unexpectedly replace the other at any time.

He is still frightened of being poisoned at the bar where he has lunch and is always ready to draw conclusions from banal events that prove there are conspiracy plots against him. Once, I crossed paths with him when he was sitting in a bar near my studio, but, since I didn't see him, I didn't greet him. In the following session, after a great deal of effort and with considerable anxiety, Giovanni confesses that he saw me: it had looked as though I was running; he was sure that I was going to a small restaurant nearby of the same nationality as his rival, which is the den of his persecutors who want him dead.

This type of communication immediately alarms me greatly: dashing hopes that the place of analysis remains unscathed from persecution, I fear I have been included in his delusion and that I may lose my analytic function. So I ask Giovanni how on earth he could believe that I, the person who is treating him, could ever think of betraying him, allying myself with the people he feels persecuted by.

Giovanni says that he knows nothing about me; I am a stranger who might betray him. For example, he adds, I might be frightened by his omnipotent persecutors, or I might be attracted by the huge sums of money they can offer me.

In the following sessions he repeats that he does not know me, the analyst, he knows nothing about me: everyone, except his parents, could be bought by his powerful enemy or be brainwashed into destroying him.

* * *

Subsequent sessions further an initial working through of this point. The patient begins to admit that, if he had the courage to investigate me, the analyst, he might think of me as a human being and so be able to step back from the image of me as a marionette without affects to be manipulated by his enemies, as suggested to him by a delusional internal voice. This acquisition could help him to construct a good relationship and to make a firm experience of it in his inner world.

I realise that the construction of the psychotic transference contains in embryonic form the same mechanism that structures the delusional system: when Giovanni feels that I am enslaved by his powerful enemies, it is obvious that he projects into me his past positions and anxieties (his being won over by power and wealth or his submission to powerful people).

I asked myself afterwards why in that session I had not interpreted to the patient that I had been transformed into a persecutor thanks to his projections; I had evidently intuited that Giovanni was incapable of understanding this type of interpretation (description of the projective identification) because his thinking was too concrete. That is why I had replied in my turn with a question that implied the possibility of going back to reflect on the psychotic transformation that had just occurred.

In that critical moment, I had realised that a dynamic interpretation would not have reached the patient because he was quite lacking any faculty for self-observation. Instead, asking him how I had become his persecutor aimed to help him go back over the chain of thoughts with which he had constructed the delusion.

Once the projection of the delusion occurred, the persecutory anxiety reached a traumatic level: the persecution was a concrete fact and everything pointed to the therapy being broken off.

My feelings of alarm stemmed from the danger *the analytic relationship* ran, the only one capable of containing the psychotic functioning and of distinguishing the healthy part from the psychotic part.

In this case, the analytic technique was based on the attempt to get the patient to recognise the elements with which he had constructed the delusion that had incorporated the figure of the analyst. As the patient recognised in the discussion following the episode, one of the elements that had encouraged the psychotic transference was certainly the quite unexpected fact of having come across me in the street. His claim to an omnipotent control of reality had been undermined and he had been left gripped by anxiety.

In that moment, the patient had not been able to distinguish the person (the analyst) from his persecutory world. In the analytic relationship, in fact, he had not progressed much and the analyst, after several months of analysis, occupied a pretty uncertain and confused position in his mind.

The interpretative technique used in this case was directed at understanding the dynamics of the delusional construction: it included descriptive interpretations that attempted to highlight the actions of the psychotic part, which presents itself to the patient as a protector but which, at the same time, sheds bad light on the objects (the analyst) that serve for good dependence. The analysis of the psychotic transference in this case progressed hand in hand with the analysis of the delusion.

Rosenfeld (1997) postulates the need for understanding the development of the psychotic transference right from the very beginning in order to prevent the delusional part from rapidly colonising the healthy part. In this case, any contamination of the analytic relationship and any compromising of the setting can become irreversible.

It is easier to contain the psychotic transference in time when the patient, as in Giovanni's case, does not conceal the delusional activity from the analyst. The situation becomes much more complex when the patient keeps his inclination for a delusional transference secret, as in the following case.

The secret delusional transference

We can talk of delusional "daydreaming" when we find ourselves in front of fantasies that have been secretly cultivated and that exist alongside, or are preserved in parallel to, the relational reality of the individual in his everyday life. However, it is possible that, at a certain point, the balance between the two realities shifts in favour of the reality constructed in the imagination.

The delusional state can be seen as a falsification worked by the imagination, of which the patient is unaware, that imposes itself on consciousness, creating a progressive distortion of reality. While the psychic reality is full of doubts, the delusional sensory reality is incontrovertible.

In Chapter Nine, I described Maria, who developed a loving transference with me. That was a singular case due to a particular element. It was not, in fact, a pre-existing delusional state that incorporated the figure of the analyst, as in Giovanni's case that I have just illustrated: the delusion, instead, emerged centred on the figure of the analyst who has to confirm the delusional desire.

Comparing the two psychotic transferences of Giovanni and Maria, we can say that while the persecutory delusional transference (such as Giovanni's) manifests itself more easily because a part of the patient wants to be freed from his anxiety, in Maria's case, the loving transference remained secret and was not communicated because she wanted to remain in the pleasurable state. In fact, Maria is seeking exhilaration and finds it in unreality by creating a fantasy situation that she claims is true.

What becomes of the analyst in the psychotic transference?

Generally, an improvement in analysis is accompanied by a progressive interiorising of the analytic function and of the figure of the analyst, something that becomes clear also in the content of the dreams from an advanced stage of analysis. In these dreams, the analyst is represented as a friendly or loving figure invested with positive emotions. During the psychotic evolution, this process of introjection suffers an arrest and a catastrophic collapse. The following clinical vignette illustrates this point.

*   *   *

While he was coming out of a megalomaniac psychotic state, a young patient brought a dream in which the representation of the attack on the analyst and on the parental couple that had been carried out during the psychotic transformation could be seen afterwards.

> In the dream, he had been invited to the home of a couple of analysts who allowed him to get into their double bed. Here he aroused himself with a series of whirling movements and reached a blissful state of pleasure. His parents appeared, washed out and far away. At a certain point, he was surrounded by deformed dachshunds with their heads stuck on backwards, that were complaining, accusing him of being responsible for their deformities.

*   *   *

The patient said that he felt that the small deformed animals in his dream were something to do with him and were like his small selves. The patient had visualised in the dream the state of masturbatory pleasure that had sustained his entrance into the delusion of omnipotence, but now he was aware of the destructive quality of this process, responsible for producing mental injury and for weakening his parents and the analyst. In the transference, the pair of analysts had allowed him to get into their bed and produce megalomaniac arousal. So, the figures of his parents appeared uncertain and washed out and, at the same time, he felt accused of having caused irreparable damage to his self.

I now report part of the material of a case in supervision that shows what happens to the figure of the analyst when the psychotic state conquers the patient's mind.

> Angela is a young woman aged twenty-one whose first psychotic episode occurred when she was sixteen with a mystic delusion and with a state of exaltation that led her to confess to having had sexual relations with Jesus Christ.[22] She had been a timid child, withdrawn in her fantasy world. After about two years of therapy, a second psychotic episode occurred in which the patient says she is the devil and begs the (female) therapist not to look her in the eyes as she is frightened of contaminating her. The crisis is dealt with at home with the help of a psychiatrist. Angela's seriously ill state means that several sessions are missed due to her being terrified of going out of the house for fear of being killed. The therapist reflected at great length on the reasons for the new crisis and discussed it in supervision.

> The supervisor's opinion is that the therapist worked too much on a symbolical level (interpretations of content) and was excessively worried

about the patient, to such an extent that sometimes not even the times of the setting were rigidly adhered to. Perhaps the anxiety that the patient transmitted to her prevented her from perceiving the specific aspects of the psychotic transformation and of containing them in time.

It was suggested to the therapist that she attempt to understand how Angela goes into the delusion and to note every communication regarding this. The patient goes to an art school and, thanks to her skill in drawing, has always been thought of as a little genius by her family. She often brought her drawings to the sessions and their content was commented on. The analytic sequence I report follows Angela's partial recovery from the psychotic episode and her regular resumption of sessions. This is the moment in which it is possible to help the patient understand the attraction that the psychosis exercises over her mind. In this sequence, Angela demonstrates a particular intuitive capacity about this point.

In a session, she speaks of a dream: "I'm in a train with my father; it's evening. We have to go to a small village nearby and, since it's evening, I imagine we will not return home that night. During the journey my father worked on his papers, very focused, and I felt a bit uncomfortable, alone. Then I'm in another car, me and my father with Mrs Franzoni[23] driving. I recognise Mrs Franzoni and feel hugely ill at ease at being in the same car as her. I get to a college, surrounded by a high wall. It's a school where they teach archery. That evening I'm in a dorm with other girls, and in the dark I see a girl smiling at me in a strange way and she's got a sort of phosphorescent bow. The next morning we all go to the swimming pool and, for fear that someone might steal my bathrobe, I swim 'doggy paddle', holding the robe above the water in my hands."

The connections the patient makes with the dream are that when she goes to the public swimming pool she is afraid that someone will take something away from her; in fact, she puts the towel and keys to the locker on the edge of the pool. When the therapist suggests that the bathrobe is like a skin, she confirms that she is afraid of losing her identity. Then she talks about the bow and says she was surprised by that girl's smile; it's the kind of smile that in fact instils fear, too. Certainly, her fear of being killed is part of it all, therefore the fact that the bow is phosphorescent is something good that can be recognised and seen.

The session comes to an end and the therapist says goodbye to the patient, saying that they both have the task of thinking about that dream.

In the next session, perhaps for the first time during her therapy, Angela brings her own worked-through contribution. She has thought a lot about what the bow in the dream might mean; for her it evoked light and so angels and demons came to mind. The analyst points out that this is the delusional part, which strikes her, enlightens and seduces her, making her believe that it is the only path for becoming something superior, an angel. The patient agrees and says that she feels she is an angel that can always become a devil.

The dream illustrates the enchantment of sensual grandiosity that has ensnared the patient, but underlines also, with great precision, that the psychotic transformation occurred through taking advantage of the father's mental absence.

We may conjecture that the mentally absent parent could also be the analyst, who did not foresee the development of the flight into delusion. In fact, in the dreams that precede or follow the psychotic state, the analyst is often represented as a colourless or mentally absent figure, while the patient is shown intent on violating universal order and on constructing a parallel reality in which she can do whatever she wants. This is allowed her thanks to the mental absence of her parents and analyst, an event that is also anamnestic, which is quite common in many psychopathological vicissitudes of psychotic patients. The patient's active position in taking advantage of the analyst's mental absence to let herself be lured by the delusional state is an important dynamic. In the college scene, a place set apart from the world in which archery is taught, Angela describes the exhilarating sensory attraction of the delusion, the sensual phosphorescent bow.

In successfully illustrating her hallucinatory reality in the dream, the patient permits the analyst to enter into her psychotic retreat.

The precise description of the weakness of the healthy part represents, I believe, the dynamic nucleus that must constantly be held in mind with all its implications throughout the course of the therapy.

The pseudo-neurotic transference in the psychotic state

It becomes more difficult to avoid the onset of a psychotic crisis during treatment when the analyst works on the patient's neurotic level and neglects the risk of a psychotic crisis.

If, on the one hand, we must expect and fear the development of a psychotic transference, a transference of a neurotic type can be present during a psychotic patient's therapy. This transference may be a defensive manoeuvre by the patient, who tends to use his pseudo-neurotic part to remove the psychotic nucleus from analysis. Indeed, at the beginning of therapy, psychotic patients frequently try to achieve a pseudo-recovery, restoring the fragile balance that had characterised their personality before the crisis. It is obvious that, in cases like these, the analyst contributes to this misunderstanding when, as in the case that follows, he conceals the pathogenic potential of the psychotic nucleus from himself and puts himself in the comforting position of not having to deal with it any more during the analytic process.

*   *   *

Ada[24] is a young woman of twenty-three. At high school she had anxiety attacks and periods of isolation, anorexia, and diets followed with obsessive severity. She was sent to analysis by a psychiatrist who had treated her during a hospital admission of several weeks, following a bizarre attempt to ingest objects that was thwarted by her mother, who had intervened, thus preventing Ada from suffocating.

At the beginning of analysis Ada feels afflicted by a sensation of emptiness and abulia, but says that before she was admitted to hospital she felt very intelligent, lucid, and creative, and was immersed in reading the great writers, especially Virginia Woolf.

In a crescendo of mental arousal, the idea had come to her that she was Lucifer, the bringer of light, the preferred angel of God. After this she had felt demonic, a bearer of all the evils in the world, and had understood that she had to kill herself in order to avert an imminent world's end.

Finally, she suddenly lost her mental lucidity. Although anxiety ridden, the state of arousal of the psychotic episode seems to constitute a special, extraordinary condition in her mind, remembered with yearning.

Therapy can be divided into two parts: in the first, anxieties prevail without psychotic symptoms; in the second, the patient returns to being psychotic.

During the first year of treatment, in fact, the material from the sessions sheds light on depressive anxiety and the collapse of identity. The analysis seemed to be progressing well and the transference interpretations, especially those regarding the analyst's feared incapacity to understand and sustain her, succeed in temporarily helping her to overcome the various moments of emptiness and anxiety.

Even if the analysis is proceeding well, one could get the impression that things were going "too" well and perhaps it would be possible to think that Ada, as far as any improvement goes, is attempting a flight towards recovery.

In any case, the analyst, convinced she had paid sufficient attention to the material, was surprised by the new psychotic episode, which began after the patient finally agreed to her father's insistent request that they go on a trip together.

*   *   *

This is why Ada misses a week of sessions. During the trip she is again ill, and delusionally thinks she is sexually aroused by her father, who would be the devil. The trip is interrupted and the patient is once again hospitalised. The virulence with which the new psychotic symptomatology erupts allows us to see how all the analytic work that one thought had been achieved is demolished in the blink of an eye. At this point, the analyst asks herself how she could have missed noticing such a deeply ingrained and unchanged persistence of the psychotic situation.

*   *   *

Evidently, up to this point, only the neurotic aspects, anxieties, and relative transference projections had been considered and the analysis had not allowed deeper penetration into the psychotic functioning, which continued to exist and exert power over the patient.

On resuming analysis, Ada says she experienced the trip with her father as an incestuous event. It seemed indecent for her and her father to be there, in a group of couples. The others took them for husband and wife on their honeymoon. And the double bedroom they slept in seemed to her like a huge red vagina that provoked her to have "sinful" thoughts towards her father.

During the psychotic episode, she was terrified of analysis and the analyst; she thought the analyst was angry with her because she had violated some rule or because she had destroyed her brain. In fact, in the preceding months, the patient had already let slip every now and then that she had got into the analyst's thoughts.

That interruption in the analysis signified a dramatic break in which the preceding psychotic episode was repeated. In the new delusional episode, it seems as though the patient acted out, through the incestuous flight with her father, an attack against the analyst-mother who had been transformed into a damaged and vindictive figure. This is why the patient felt guilty and threatened by the analyst, who represents the persecutory psychotic superego.

At the peak of this destructive atmosphere, Ada felt diabolical (as in the first episode in which she was Lucifer), in league with the figure of her father, who also represents part of her, the part that pushes her to project herself into a manic sexualised reality.

*   *   *

Facing up to the new psychotic episode, the analyst, who had under-estimated the danger of a new psychotic crisis, understands that she had arrived "afterwards", when the psychic catastrophe had already been produced.

Not having been able to oppose her father's wish (which had soun-ded like an ultimatum to the patient), Ada must have put the analyst in the position of a weak mother who is swept away by the sexualised father.

Two dreams, which precede the crisis and whose significance can only be recognised now, refer back to the eroticisation of the feared father figure, which is then manifested in the delusional explosion:

> "We are in the mountains, skiing; in the evening we have to go to our rooms. I hope I will be in the room of a boy I fancy but unfortunately I've drawn Father X, who is an Italian teacher. He wants to touch me; I run away; he pursues me; the house dissolves into a castle. Wherever I go, fires break out . . ."

> "At home my parents are having an orgy; they are like drunks, people jumping on the beds. My parents enjoy seeing me arrive at that point. I'm mad at them, I try to get my creams and make-up. But I can't; it's as though I was hanging, my hands are busy, as in a porn film."

In these dreams, Ada describes how she can create, by transform-ing her parents into perverse objects, an orgiastic state of mind with the resulting entrapment of herself in a sexualised world. Her impris-onment in the psychosis and her total loss of any perception of human relationships derive from her acquiescence ("it's as though I was hang-ing, my hands are busy").

Despite all the possible limitations that derive from the complexity this treatment has assumed, this patient's dreams became a privileged vehicle for understanding the altered mental states, even before they were clinically manifested.

Understanding them aided the construction of an analytic relationship that laid the foundations for preventing and avoiding further psychotic implosions because the analyst had become more capable of seeing the psychosis being prepared in the dream. In Ada's case, it was important to understand that the neurotic transference, carried on throughout the whole of the first year of analysis with the tacit agreement of the analyst, was afterwards revealed to be a defence against a potential psychotic transformation that was always lying in wait. Therefore, as I have said above, there was reciprocal collusion between patient and analyst, seeing that the latter underestimated the psychotic episode that had occurred before analysis and had not worked on that.

A further observation about collusion must be made concerning the father's role in the patient's analysis. The father, a successful man with a grandiose, manic character, did not think very favourably about his daughter's analysis and, in fact, had obtained her agreement to go on holiday with him without considering the problem of her missing sessions. Unexpected interference by relatives in the analysis of psychotics is not infrequent. But, at a deeper level, Ada adheres to the manic father who prefers to go on holiday with her rather than with her mother. It is by no means rare for psychotic patients to identify, from early infancy, with the pathological aspects of one or both parents.

In Ada's inner world, the transformation of the figure of the analyst into an aggressive vindictive figure who wants to punish her stems from the eroticised fusion with her father.

An internal object that pushes towards madness

In some cases, the dreams of psychotic patients are very useful because they describe extremely clearly the dynamics of the psychotic nucleus in relation to other parts of the personality. I believe that it is very important, in these cases, to give the patient descriptive interpretations, when the material allows, so that action by the psychotic part can be contained and isolated. Particular attention must be paid to the intrapsychic dynamics between the psychotic part and the non-psychotic part of the personality.

I discuss this problem, taking my cue from one of Ada's dreams:

> "I am at an exhibition of Dalí's work. There is an empty antechamber with columns like the giraffe-necks of Dalí's women. I ask Dalí to accompany me into a room because I'm afraid. He comes into another room with me and gives me a piece of the Madonna sculpture to eat, on which is written 'it's too late by now'. I ask him to take me home because I don't have the car keys. The car changes into a treadmill, it goes up, it's like an elastic band that you have to pull with both hands. It's very steep; I laugh like a mad thing and throw myself backwards."

This dream could be interpreted as a transferral dream: the character of Dalí could be taken for the analyst who wields such attraction over her that it takes her outside reality into a surreal world. It is, in fact, possible that the patient has projected her madness into the analyst so that it is no longer indistinguishable from her mad part.

Yet, in this case, it seems to me that there are no elements signalling that we are facing a possible delusional transference. Rather, we are facing a dream that clearly describes the conquering action of the psychotic part (the Surrealist painter) over the healthy part.

An interpretation centred on the analyst would be confusing for the patient, who might perceive it as if the analyst was saying to her that she (analyst) is the character in the dream that wants to arouse her and make her mad. In this case, the patient would respond with persecutory anxiety.

It is more useful and more correct to make an *intrapsychic* interpretation and describe how two parts of herself exist in her internal world: one part, Salvador Dalí, who wants to win her over, arousing her and making her believe she is a great artist, but who, in fact, deceives her and makes her mad, and another part which yields to the attraction of the first. (Ada, in fact, had already spoken of her attraction to Dalí's painting and to Surrealism, to automatic writing that "frees the unconscious", and to mental logorrhea, and in the past had had periods of graphomania during which she scribbled away for days and days.)

The dream with Salvador Dalí (the Surrealist painter who transformed reality) is strongly indicative of the psychotic part's seductive action that, this time, is portrayed and communicated to the analyst.

The interpretation on an intrapsychic level of this dream was particularly significant because it allowed the patient's participation in the construction of the psychotic state that led to her first hospital admission to emerge. Naturally, this type of approach is connected to the model that distinguishes the psychotic part from the neurotic part and explains the psychotic crisis as the conquest of the first over the second.

Descriptive interpretations centred on the inner world are capable of helping the patient understand and differentiate healthy objects that aid development from psychotic ones that drive it to madness.

Dreaming the transference

To explain the difference between the neurotic and the psychotic transference, I will make use of an analogy between transference and dream based on Bion's affirmation (1959, 1992) that psychotic patients are incapable of "dreaming". The transference has many similarities with dreams: for example, it contains a meaning that is not manifest that the analyst can interpret; furthermore, unconscious activity that emotionally invests another subject, the analyst, is needed for a transference to be established.

In the neurotic transference, the repressed reality and the conscious one are both present and are projected into the analyst who, as a transferral object, holds an "as if" position, halfway between fantasy and reality. The analogy between the structure of the dream and that of the transference would also explain why the neurotic patient remains in a position full of doubts, and accepts the interpretation of the transference as though it were that of the dream. It is, therefore, possible to posit that neurotic patients are able to "dream" the transference, and, thus, to create it, while patients in the psychotic state cannot do so.

Lying at the origin of the development of a psychotic transference are not so much the processes of repressing the emotional past and projection, but, rather, vertical splits between the psychotic nucleus and the rest of the personality.

In the psychotic state the transference loses its "dream" quality because the capacity to symbolise is lost. The symbolical interpretation of the transference is experienced by the psychotic patient as the revelation of another factual reality, and not as a repressed reality.

In Ada's case, if the analyst had given her a transferral inter-pretation, the patient would have perceived that the analyst really was Salvador Dalí, with all the arousing implications and connected anxieties.

What is transferred?

Referring to the nature of the psychotic transference and to its poten-tial for transforming, I maintain that the delusional production is transferred in the psychotic transference, whereas childhood issues (Freud) or the unconscious parts of the personality (Klein) are trans-ferred in the normal transference.

So, a transformative activity of reality is transferred "into the present", rather than a truth from the past. An altered perception of the figure of the analyst also exists in the normal transference, but this distortion depends on the repression of the past or on a non-aware-ness of parts of the self that are projected.

The neurotic transference moves from the dynamic unconscious, which has its roots in childhood, whereas the psychotic transference is produced by the psychotic functioning and has no connection with the childhood past. It is a hyper-saturated, concrete space, a "dead point" incapable of evolution. It could be indicated by the capital letter T preceded by the minus sign: $-T$.

In an apparently paradoxical way, we can state that in the usual analytic process we hope that the sick nucleus will enter the transfer-ence so that it can be worked through, whereas in psychosis the production of the psychotic transference does not serve the therapy at all; on the contrary, it bears witness to the fact that the uncontained psychotic activity has spilled over into a space that has to be kept free. In the light of what we have said, and taking up Rosenfeld's proposi-tion (1997) that the psychotic transference must be transformed as quickly as possible, we can also affirm that it is necessary to work ana-lytically to prevent this event from happening.

We must help the patient find a way out by working from the delu-sional world, dissociated from reality, restoring him to a way of func-tioning in which the laws of psychic reality and of emotional bonds are accepted and deemed indispensable for psychic survival.

CHAPTER NINETEEN

Difficult patients: conclusions

I start out from the premise that the analyst who treats difficult patients should have in mind the entire field of mental suffering (from neurosis to psychosis) and should be conversant with the path and pathogenic evolution of the individual illnesses.

The cases presented in this book illustrate the nosographic categories that move within precise coordinates and, as such, require a specific therapeutic approach.

I have explored several pathologies that I believe are difficult to transform and that require a particular creative effort from analytic technique and theory. Naturally, I have not been able to consider all cases that are difficult, which, sometimes, go beyond our actual capacities. An example of this is anorexia in its pure form. There we witness the mind truly disappearing into the body and prevailing behaviours released from every psychological context that testify to a profound split between body and emotions.

A number of very difficult patients live in constant dread of being overwhelmed by unbearable pain. We are all too familiar with the mechanisms that are brought into play in the attempt to emerge from this desperate situation: alcohol abuse, drug addiction, compulsive sexuality, arousing fantasies, and so on.

When something traumatic occurs during the earliest phases of the self's structuring, a nucleus of dark, silent suffering is created. When the pain reaches an unbearable peak, the desire to die (with all its dramatic consequences) seems to be the only way to put an end to such agony. In this case, the eventual suicide serves to break the vicious circle of pain; it does not have the same aggressive or vindictive significance as that of a melancholic's.

During analysis, these patients are, for the most part, passive, ready to emotively vanish if the analyst is not mentally alert, always present, and willing to participate. With them, we must reawaken their vitality and the capacity to bind themselves to objects they can usefully depend on.

Naturally the ability to experience good dependence differs from individual to individual and depends on whether psychopathological structures working against the possibility of establishing bonds that aid emotional development are present or not.

An example of the former are those patients who have constructed pathological structures (perverse, borderline, or psychotic) that they shut themselves up in. The sensitive and alive part of their personality has both suffered an arrest and been profoundly damaged, as it is held prisoner by the pathological process. We have to work long and hard to strip the distorting structures dominating the patient of their power before it is possible to try and nurture this part.

The difficulty in treatment, in fact, depends on the quantity and quality of the psychopathological structures that the patient has generated in alliance, sometimes, with his original environment. Some of these structures are potentially extremely dangerous because they tend to engulf and destroy the entire personality.

The transference and its interpretation are two important elements to consider with regard to the analytic technique in the therapy of difficult patients.

In Chapter Eighteen, I describe the danger of the psychotic transference contaminating the analytic relationship and effectively halting the developmental process. In general, it can be said that it is not a positive sign when the patient includes the analyst in his psychopathological structure. For example, a perverse patient may include the analyst in his perverse fantasies in order to use him as an object in his possession and strip him of his analytic function. This transference contamination tends to happen when the analyst has not shown himself capable of bringing the sick parts of the patient into focus.

I believe that the psychopathological structure must remain outside the transference for it to be worked through. Interpretations must concentrate—with great tenacity, delicacy, and attention—in the first place on describing the power wielded by the pathological organisations.

In the clinical cases presented, psychic withdrawal, variously structured, is a constant element: of a sexualised nature in the perversions, fantastic in the borderlines, delinquent in destructive narcissism, confusing and destructive in the structures that organise the psychosis. In these pages, I have frequently emphasised that the analytic work of difficult cases must concentrate on the patient's internal world and develop his healthy parts, which must progressively become aware of the nature and aims of the sick parts. The analytic treatment coincides with the opportunity for creating a relationship in which it becomes possible to nourish and enrich the patient's mind. This is why the analyst must speak to the healthy part in order to shed light on the workings of the sick part. The work required of the analyst in these cases does not often have much to do with interpreting the transference, although, naturally, when this is present it must be interpreted.

Freud originally postulated that the neurosis originated from an infant complex and that during therapy this complex was transferred to the figure of the analyst. Through interpreting the transference, the analyst helped the patient to distinguish himself from the past object. In its turn, knowledge of the past encouraged a reconstruction of the childhood story and released it from repression.

In the case of difficult patients, the work on their repressed past is only relatively useful, whereas the exploration of their internal world is much more important. In the first place, the interpretative work must be advanced through interpretations that focus on the internal world and on the dynamics between the healthy and sick parts. A lack of awareness of the harmful nature of the latter is one of the characteristics of difficult patients.

Human beings are not born with an apparatus for perceiving their emotions, but do possess the potential for developing it. As we have learnt from Bion, for this apparatus to develop, there must be a mother who gives suitable responses and confirms the child's emotional preconception.

I believe that difficult patients experienced an emotional deficit on the part of the their parents followed by a lack of structuring of the psyche and the ensuing development of pathogenic structures.

In this book, I discuss the emotional trauma (see, especially, Chapter Three) in order to distinguish it from an acute phenomenally evident trauma and to illustrate the pathogenic relations that in various ways (for example, through the parents' emotional absence or, in contrast, thanks to their particularly psychological intrusion) prevent the development, from infancy, of a mental structure fit for understanding psychic reality. Along the way, I refer to Bion's hypotheses (lack of the functions of containing and maternal reverie), and to Winnicott's (insufficient holding), and to Fonagy's (disorder in recognising one's individuality and sense of self).

In Chapter Seven, I maintain that the parents' psychic absence prevents the correct structuring of the *emotional unconscious*.

I find it useful to distinguish at least two meanings for the unconscious—probably corresponding to different functions of the mind—which I have called the dynamic unconscious and the emotional–receptive unconscious (Chapter Seven).

The former is the repressed unconscious, discovered by Freud, knowledge of which was further developed and expanded by Melanie Klein, who emphasised the mechanisms of splitting and projection leading to the focus on projective identification.

The latter was described by Bion, who prizes its function of the metaboliser of psychic experiences rather than of a place in which the repressed can be deposited.

These two conceptions of the unconscious do not exclude each other but are, in fact, complementary, a relationship that lends itself to being described through the metaphor of a building: the emotional unconscious represents the foundations, what lies below, understood also as below ground, and so can never be seen (never known), while the dynamic unconscious, what lies above, can be seen (and therefore known).

The emotional unconscious constantly constructs the notion of personal identity, which determines the way of relating to the world, generating the capacity to perceive and deal with emotions, defining the unaware consciousness of existing. In my opinion, the majority of difficult patients lack these characteristics.

I have advanced this distinction because I believe that there is something in difficult patients that renders the aware–unaware system, rather than the conscious–unconscious system, inactive. The majority of difficult patients, in fact, are *unaware*, especially because they do not perceive the self-destructive nature of the pathological constructions.

Acquisition of the intuitive faculty and perception of self is something that happens during the first months of life through non-verbal and unaware procedures. So, they are functions that are created at the same time as the bases of the personality are formed. Patients that are the object of my considerations in this book do not have the capacity to think emotionally because, as children, they isolated themselves in response to a deficient maternal empathy, withdrawing into an imaginary world made up of imagined sensory excitations.

A number of authors in the past, for example, Ferenczi, highlighted the role of the patient's traumatic story as the source of suffering and attempted to place the therapist in the active position of substitute object capable of repairing the original damage. In my view, the analyst already positions himself as a different object from the one in the past because he is endowed with that receptive emotional capacity that the former object was lacking.

The specific element of this therapeutic stance lies not only in accepting the patient's traumatic suffering, but also in working on the structures that arose from the trauma and that are still active and at work. In other words, it is necessary to work on what the patient himself has contributed and continues to contribute to his disorder.

This is why, when we get into the essentials of therapy, I propose we should carry out our work by way of *deconstructions*, or *descriptive* interpretations capable of helping the patient to understand his own internal world and to differentiate the objects that help his development from those that damage it, rather than by way of interpretations of meaning. While interpretations of content refer to the symbolic level, deconstruction involves gradually recognising how the pathogenic nucleus was built up and developed, through examining the emotional conditions both present and past preparatory to the disorder.

Difficult patients were children deprived of an experience capable of structuring their minds and this deprivation facilitated their withdrawal into a world apart.

Three different groups belong to this category of patients: the perverse, the borderline, and the psychotic. Psychic withdrawal has played an important role for all of them. However, the state of arousal and sexualised fantasies present in the perversions do not interfere, to any great degree, with the bond with reality or with the functions of thought. Psychosis, however, wields huge destructive potential because it annihilates—sometimes irreversibly—the foundations of personality. The perverse subject distorts the rules of human relations; the psychotic distorts and destroys the rules of thought themselves.

Difficult patients cannot avail themselves of symbolic thought: they have related for such a long time to fantasy sensory objects and so have only the experience of a concrete reality. When these patients come out of the psychopathological state and come into contact with psychic reality, they are disorientated and confused; they realise then that there is an unknown world that they have never lived in and do not know.

As I have attempted to show, in my analytic work with difficult patients I focus on exploring their internal world, their traumatic story, and, especially, the effects that the intrusive childhood objects have had on the construction of psychopathological structures. In other words, I try to go beyond the transference and the counter-transference, which, when they exist, should be used and trans-formed.

I believe that the analyst must constantly integrate the patient's world with all the elements (memories, reconstructions, reflections on experiences of life, including those of the analyst) that may be useful for expanding the patient's psychic life.

For difficult patients, too, the therapeutic result depends on the analyst's skill in creating a specific place in his mind for the analysand (for his story, his problems, and his tacit demands for mental and emotional development) and on the patient's readiness to consider the analyst a transformative object that is indispensable for his growth. The analytic process continues and progresses as long as this intimate and creative relationship remains alive, allowing the patient to learn about emotional reality and to discover his own personal significance.

In this book, I have attempted to clarify the nature and origin of some conditions of illness, and I have endeavoured to build what we may call a psychoanalytic psychopathology. In fact, I do not believe it is possible to prepare any effective therapeutic tool before knowing the nature of the disorder and the path by which the patient arrives at that state of illness. I am convinced that there is still much to be done for difficult patients, in both the theoretical field and the clinical field, and I hope that this book will be followed by other contributions that, in holding psychoanalysis firmly anchored to clinical work, will lead to the successful treatment of the many cases otherwise lost along wrong paths and destined never to recover from their ill state.

1. I discussed this case with Dr Paola Capozzi.
2. The hippocampus is made up of a set of neurons that are found bilaterally in the depth of the parietal lobes. The amygdala is a small globe-like formation sited in the medial part of the temporal lobe. LeDoux (1996) describes how the amygdala coordinates and activates the primitive circuit of fear (see also "panic attacks" in Chapter Ten).
3. I discussed this case with Dr Giorgio Mattana.
4. This material was presented to me in supervision by Dr Maria Grazia Gallo.
5. These brief introductory notes are taken from my earlier historical–critical discussion of the superego (De Masi, 1989).
6. During the analysis, a strongly censored memory emerged that she had been the object of sexual attentions by her father when she was young. The censorship was partly due to her feeling that she was to blame for what had occurred. She subsequently learnt that the same had happened to her younger sister.
7. This case will be described more fully in Chapter Ten.
8. Compare with the patient described earlier who was dependent on the boy-idol.
9. This brief summary of the models of the unconscious of Freud, Klein, and Bion is taken from my book *Vulnerability to Psychosis* (De Masi, 2009[2006]).

10. Criticism of Green's thesis is expressed in an article by Trevor Lubbe (2008), in which the author not only takes up Klein's idea, but also emphasises the importance of sexuality in the work of Donald Meltzer.

11. This division can be found in my book *The Sadomasochistic Perversion. The Entity and the Theories* (De Masi, 2003[1999]).

12. According to Sulloway (1979), this version has become something of a myth, not only because it was actually Anna O who broke off the therapy, but also on account of documentary evidence that the birth of Breuer's daughter, supposedly conceived on his second honeymoon, predated the patient's loving transference.

13. See Kerr (1993) for a fascinating account of the events concerned and of the relations between Freud, Jung, and Sabina.

14. I discussed this material, which corresponds to two interviews with a child whose parents decided not to accept the proposal of psychoanalytic treatment for their son, with Dr Manuela Moriggia.

15. This case was brought to me in supervision by Dr Rossana Russo.

16. This case, following psychoanalytic therapy at two sessions a week, was presented to me by Dr Francesco Comelli.

17. Instead, Professor Paolo Valerio believes that some transsexuals openly manifest a desire for maternity (personal communication). A similar statement was made to me by Dr Maurizio Bini, the head of Gynaecology at the Niguarda Hospital in Milan.

18. This case was discussed in supervision with a colleague, Franziska Henningsen of Berlin.

19. In some languages, for example French, there is only one word for the two terms "unconscious" and "unaware".

20. This material was given to me by Dr Rossana Russo.

21. 1 I have already described this patient, also mentioned in Chapter Seventeen, in my book *Vulnerability to Psychosis* (2009[2006]).

22. The patient was followed by Dr Marina Medioli.

23. Anna Maria Franzoni is an Italian mother convicted of infanticide.

24. I discussed this case with Dr Paola Capozzi. The same material is present in Capozzi and De Masi (2001).

REFERENCES

Abraham, K. (1973[1907]). The experiencing of sexual trauma as a form of sexual activity. In: *Selected Papers on Psycho-Analysis* (pp. 47–63). London: Hogarth.

Abraham, K. (1973[1924]). A short study of the development of the libido, viewed in the light of mental disorders. In: *Selected Papers on Psycho-Analysis* (pp. 418–501). London: Hogarth.

Adler, G. (1988). How useful is the borderline concept? *Psychoanalytic Inquiry, 8*: 353–372.

Amati-Mehler, J. (1984). Riflessioni sul "bambino tecnologico". *Rivista di Psicoanalisi, 2*: 299–306.

Anders, G. (1985). Die Antiquiertheit des Hassens. In: R. Kahle, H. Menzner, & G. Vinnai (Eds.), *Hass. Die Macht eines unerwünschten Gefühls* (pp. 11–32). Reinbek bei Hamburg: Rowohlt.

Anzieu, D., & Monjauze, M. (2004). *Francis Bacon. Ou le portrait de l'homme désespécé*. Paris: Seuil-Archimbaud.

Argentieri, S. (2006). Travestitismo, transessualismo, transgender: identificazione e imitazione. *Psicoanalisi, 2*: 55–91.

Arundale, J. (1999). Notes on a case of paedophilia. In: S. Ruszczynsky & S. Johnson (Eds.), *Psychoanalytic Psychotherapy in the Kleinian Tradition* (pp. 135–152). London: Karnac.

Badaracco, J. G. (1983). Reflexiones sobre sueño y psicosis a la luz de la experiencia clínica. *Revista de Psicoanálisis, 40*, 4: 693–709.

Balint, M. (1956). Perversions and procreation. In: S. Lorand & M. Balint (Eds.), *Perversions. Psychodynamics and Therapy*. New York: Random House.

Balint, M. (1968). *The Basic Fault. Therapeutic Aspects of Regression*. London: Tavistock.

Barrie, J. M. (1995). *Peter Pan and Other Plays*. Oxford: Clarendon (World's Classics).

Bataille, G. (2001[1961]). *The Tears of Eros*, P. Connor (Trans.). San Francisco, CA: City Lights.

Baudrillard, J. (1999). *Il virtuale ha assorbito il reale. Intervista a Jean Baudrillard*, In: MediaMente (www.mediamente.rai.it/home/bibliote/intervis/b/baudrillard.htm) accessed on 28 December 2013.

Beebe, B., Lachmann, F., & Jaffe, J. (1997). Mother–infant structures and presymbolic self and object representation. *Psychoanalytic Dialogues, 7*: 133–182.

Bion, W. R. (1957). Differentiation of the psychotic from the non-psychotic personalities. *International Journal of Psychoanalysis, 38*: 266–275.

Bion, W. R. (1959). *Second Thoughts*. London: Heinemann.

Bion, W. R. (1962). *Learning from Experience*. London: Heinemann.

Bion, W. R. (1970). *Attention and Interpretation. A Scientific Approach to Insight in Psycho-Analysis*. London: Tavistock.

Bion, W. R. (1978). *Four Discussions with W. R. Bion*. Strathtay, Perthshire: Clunie Press.

Bion, W. R. (1992). *Cogitations*, F. Bion (Ed.). London: Karnac.

Bleichmar, H. (2004). Making conscious the unconscious in order to modify unconscious processing. Some mechanisms of therapeutic change. *International Journal of Psychoanalysis, 85*: 1379–1400.

Blum, H. P. (1973). The concept of erotized transference. *Journal of the American Psychoanalytic Association, 21*: 61–76.

Bollas, C. (1979). The transformational object. *International Journal of Psychoanalysis, 60*: 97–107.

Bollas, C. (1987). *The Shadow of the Object. Psychoanalysis of the Unthought Known*. London: Free Association.

Bollas, C. (1989). *Forces of Destiny. Psychoanalysis and Human Idiom*. London: Free Association.

Bollas, C. (1992). *Being a Character. Psychoanalysis and Self Experience*. New York: Farrar, Strauss & Giroux.

Bollas, C. (1995). *Cracking Up*. New York: Hill & Wang.

Bollas, C. (2009). *The Infinite Question*. London: Routledge.

Bolognini, S. (1994). Transference: erotised, erotic, loving, affectionate. *International Journal of Psychoanalysis, 75*: 73–86.

Bordi, S. (2009). *Scritti.* Milan: Cortina.

Brenman, E. (2002). Matters of life and death – real and assumed. In: *Recovery of the Lost Good Object* (pp. 34–47). London: Routledge.

Brenman, E. (2006). *Recovery of the Lost Good Object.* London: Routledge.

Briggs, J. (1986). Expecting the unexpected. Canadian Inuit training for an experimental life-style. Paper delivered to the IV International Conference on Hunting and Gathering Societies. London School of Economics.

Busch de Ahumada, L. C. (2003). Clinical notes on a case of transvestism in a child. *International Journal of Psychoanalysis, 84:* 291–313.

Bychowski, G. (1966). Psychosis precipitated by psychoanalysis. *Psychoanalytic Quarterly, 35:* 327–339.

Cantarella, E. (1992). *Bisexuality in the Ancient World.* New Haven, CT: Yale University Press.

Caper, R. (1998). Psychopathology and primitive mental states. *International Journal of Psychoanalysis, 79:* 539–551.

Capozzi, P., & De Masi, F. (2001). The meaning of dreams in the psychotic states: theoretical considerations and clinical applications. *International Journal of Psychoanalysis, 82:* 933–952.

Carey, B. (2008). Standing in someone else's shoes, almost for real. *The New York Times,* 1 December, p. D5.

Carotenuto, A. (1982). *A Secret Symmetry. Sabina Spielrein between Jung and Freud.* New York: Pantheon Books.

Carrara, S., & Zanda, G. (2008). Conference on "La psiche nella rete: Nuove opportunità e nuove patologie", Lucca, Italy, 15 November. In: *Psicoanalisi e metodo, 9,* 2009.

Carroll, L. (1971). *Alice in Wonderland.* Oxford: Oxford University Press.

Chasseguet-Smirgel, J. (1973). Essai sur l'ideal du moi. *Revue Française de Psychanalyse, 37:* 735–910.

Chasseguet-Smirgel, J. (1985). *Creativity and Perversion.* London: Free Association.

Chiland, C. (1998). Transvestism and transsexualism. *International Journal of Psychoanalysis, 79:* 156–159.

Chiland, C. (2000). The psychoanalyst and the transsexual patient. *International Journal of Psychoanalysis, 81:* 21–35.

Chiland, C. (2004). Gender and sexual difference. In: I. Mathis (Ed.), *Dialogues on Sexuality, Gender and Psychoanalysis.* London: Karnac.

Chiland, C. (2005[1997]). *Exploring Transsexualism.* London: Karnac.

Chiland, C. (2009). Some thoughts on transsexualism, transvestism, transgender, and identification. In: G. Ambrosio (Ed.), *Transvestism, Transsexualism in the Psychoanalytic Dimension.* London: Karnac.

Chodorow, N. J. (1992). Heterosexuality as a compromise formation. Reflections on the psychoanalytic theory of sexual development. *Psychoanalysis and Contemporary Thought, 15*: 267–304.

Coates, S. (2006). Developmental research on childhood gender identity disorder. In: P. Fonagy, M. Leuzinger-Bohleber, & R. Krause (Eds.), *Identity, Gender, Sexuality. 150 Years after Freud.* London: Karnac.

Coates, S., & Moore, M. S. (1997). The complexity of early trauma. Representation and transformation. *Psychoanalytic Inquiry, 17*: 286–311.

Coates, S., Friedman, R. C., & Wolfe, S. (1991). The etiology of boyhood gender identity disorder. A model for integrating temperament, development, and psychodynamic. *Psychoanalytic Dialogues, 1*: 481–523.

Cooper, A. (2002). *Sex and the Internet.* New York: Brunner-Routledge.

Covington, C., & Wharton, B. (2003). *Sabina Spielrein: Forgotten Pioneer of Psychoanalysis.* New York: Brunner-Routledge.

Davies, J. M. (1996). Dissociation, repression, and reality testing in the countertransference. The controversy over memory and false memory in the psychoanalytic treatment of adult survivors of childhood sexual abuse. *Psychoanalytic Dialogues, 6*: 189–218.

De Masi, F. (1988). Idealizzazione ed erotizzazione nella relazione analitica. *Rivista di Psicoanalisi, 34*: 76–120.

De Masi, F. (1989). Il super-io. *Rivista di Psicoanalisi, 35*: 393–431.

De Masi, F. (1996). Strategie psichiche verso l'autoannientamento. *Rivista di Psicoanalisi, 42*: 549–566.

De Masi, F. (2003[1999]). *The Sadomasochistic Perversion: The Entity and the Theories.* London: Karnac.

De Masi, F. (2009[2006]). *Vulnerability to Psychosis: A Psychoanalytic Study of the Nature and Therapy of the Psychotic State.* London: Karnac.

Di Ceglie, D. (1998). Reflections on the nature of the "Atypical gender identity organization". In: D. Di Ceglie & D. Freedman (Eds.), *A Stranger in My Own Body: Atypical Gender Identity Development and Mental Health* (pp. 9–25). London: Karnac.

Di Ceglie, D. (2000). Gender identity disorder in young people. In: *Advances in Psychiatric Treatment.* The Royal College of Psychiatrists, 6: 458–466.

Di Ceglie, D. (2009). Between Scylla and Charybdis: exploring atypical gender identity developments in children and adolescents. In: G. Ambrosio (Ed.), *Transvestism, Transsexualism in the Psychoanalytic Dimension* (pp. 55–72). London: Karnac.

Di Chiara, G. (1985). Una prospettiva psicoanalitica del dopo Freud: un posto per l'altro. *Rivista di Psicoanalisi, 31*: 451–461.

Emde, R. N. (1989). The infant's relationship experience: developmental and affective aspects. In: A. I. Sameroff & R. N. Emde (Eds.), *Relationship Disturbances in Early Childhood: A Developmental Approach*. New York: Basic Books.

Fabbri, D. (2006). Per l'orgasmo clicca qui [Click here for orgasm]. *Io Donna*, 23 February.

Federn, P. (1952). *Ego Psychology and the Psychoses*. London: Imago, 1953.

Ferenczi, S. (1929). The unwelcome child and his death-instinct. *International Journal of Psychoanalysis, 10*: 125–129.

Ferenczi, S. (1955[1933]). Confusion of tongues between adults and the child. In: M. Balint (Ed.), *Final Contributions to the Problems and Methods of Psycho-Analysis* (pp. 102–107). London: Hogarth.

Fonagy, P. (1999). Memory and therapeutic action. *International Journal of Psychoanalysis, 80*: 215–223.

Fonagy, P. (2005). Psychoanalytic development theory. In: E. S. Person, A. M. Cooper, & G. O. Gabbard (Eds.), *The American Psychiatric Publishing Textbook of Psychoanalysis*. Washington, DC: American Publishing.

Fonagy, P. (2006). Psychoanalysis and psychosexuality: an overview. In: P. Fonagy, M. Leuzinger-Bohleber, & R. Krause (Eds.), *Identity, Gender, Sexuality. 150 Years after Freud*. London: Karnac.

Fonagy, P., & Target, M. (1996). Playing with reality: 1, Theory of mind and the normal development of psychic reality. *International Journal of Psychoanalysis, 77*: 217–233.

Fraiberg, S. (1982). Pathological defences in infancy. *Psychoanalytic Quarterly, 51*: 612–635.

Freud, A. (1961). *The Ego and the Mechanisms of Defence*. London: Hogarth and The Institute of Psycho-Analysis.

Freud, S. (1894b). The neuro-psychoses of defence. *S.E., 3*: 43–61. London: Hogarth.

Freud, S. (with J. Breuer) (1895d). *Studies on Hysteria. S.E., 2*: 1–335. London: Hogarth.

Freud, S. (1905d). *Three Essays on the Theory of Sexuality. S.E., 7*: 125–245. London: Hogarth.

Freud, S. (1905e). *Fragment of an Analysis of a Case of Hysteria. S.E., 7*: 3–112. London: Hogarth.

Freud, S. (1909b). *Analysis of a Phobia in a Five-year-old Boy. S.E., 10*: 3–251. London: Hogarth.

Freud, S. (1911c). *Psycho-analytic Notes on an Autobiographical Account of a Case of Paranoia* (dementia paranoides). *S.E.*, *12*: 3–84. London: Hogarth.

Freud, S. (1912b). The dynamics of transference. *S.E.*, *12*: 98–108. London: Hogarth.

Freud, S. (1912e). Recommendations to physicians practising psycho-analysis. *S.E.*, *12*: 111–120 London: Hogarth.

Freud, S. (1914c). On narcissism: an introduction. *S.E.*, *14*: 69–102. London: Hogarth.

Freud, S. (1915a). Observations on transference-love. *S.E.*, *12*: 157–170. London: Hogarth.

Freud, S. (1915c). Instincts and their vicissitudes. *S.E.*, *14*: 111–140. London: Hogarth.

Freud, S. (1915e). The unconscious. *S.E.*, *14*: 159–204. London: Hogarth.

Freud, S. (1917e). Mourning and melancholia. *S.E.*, *14*: 237–258. London: Hogarth.

Freud, S. (1919e). 'A child is being beaten'. *S.E.*, *17*: 175–204. London: Hogarth.

Freud, S. (1920g). *Beyond the Pleasure Principle. S.E.*, *18*: 3–64. London: Hogarth.

Freud, S. (1923b). *The Ego and the Id. S.E.*, *19*: 3–66. London: Hogarth.

Freud, S. (1924b). Neurosis and psychosis. *S.E.*, *19*: 147–153. London: Hogarth.

Freud, S. (1924c). The economic problem of masochism. *S.E.*, *19*: 157–170. London: Hogarth.

Freud, S. (1924d). The dissolution of the Oedipus complex. *S.E.*, *19*: 173–179. London: Hogarth.

Freud, S. (1924e). The loss of reality in neurosis and psychosis. *S.E. 19*: 182–187. London: Hogarth.

Freud, S. (1925j). Some psychical consequences of the anatomical distinction between the sexes. *S.E.*, *19*: 243–259. London: Hogarth.

Freud, S. (1926d). *Inhibitions, Symptoms and Anxiety. S.E.*, *20*: 77–174. London: Hogarth.

Freud, S. (1927d). Humour. *S.E.*, *21*: 160–166. London: Hogarth.

Freud, S. (1927e). Fetishism. *S.E.*, *21*: 152–158. London: Hogarth.

Freud, S. (1930a). *Civilization and Its Discontents. S.E.*, *21*: 59–145. London: Hogarth.

Freud, S. (1933a). *New Introductory Lectures on Psycho-analysis. S.E.*, *22*: 3–182. London: Hogarth.

Freud, S. (1936a). A disturbance of memory on the Acropolis. An open letter to Romain Rolland on the occasion of his seventieth birthday. *S.E.*, *22*: 239–248. London: Hogarth.

Freud, S. (1937c). Analysis terminable and interminable. *S.E.*, *23*: 211–253. London: Hogarth.

Freud, S. (1940a). *An Outline of Psycho-Analysis*, *S.E.*, *23*: 141–208. London: Hogarth.

Freud, S. (1940e). Splitting of the ego in the process of defence. *S.E.*, *23*: 273–278. London: Hogarth.

Garland, C. (2010). Psychoanalytic group therapy with severely disturbed patients: benefits and challenger. In: P. Williams (Ed.), *The Psychoanalytic Therapy of Severe Disturbance*. London: Karnac.

Giustino, G. (2009). Memory in dreams. *International Journal of Psychoanalysis*, *90*: 1057–1073.

Glasser, M. (1988). Psychodynamic aspect of paedophilia. *Psychoanalytic Psychotherapy*, *2*: 121–135.

Glasser, M. (1998). On violence: a preliminary communication. *International Journal of Psychoanalysis*, *79*: 887–902.

Glenn, J. (1984). Psychic trauma and masochism. *Journal of the American Psychoanalytic Association*, *32*: 357–386.

Gould, E. (1994). A case of erotized transference in a male patient formations and transformations. *Psychoanalytic Inquiry*, *14*: 558–571.

Green, A. (1997). Opening remarks to a discussion of sexuality in contemporary psychoanalysis. *International Journal of Psychoanalysis*, *78*: 345–350.

Green, A. (2001). The dead mother. In: *Life Narcissism, Death Narcissism*, A. Weller (Trans.). London: Free Association.

Green, A. (2011). *Illusions and Disillusions of Psychoanalytic Work*. London: Karnac.

Green, J. (1950). *If I Were You*. London: Eyre & Spottiswoode.

Grossman, W. J. (1991). Pain, aggression, fantasy and concept of sadomasochism. *Psychoanalytic Quarterly*, *40*, *19*: 22–53.

Grotstein, J. (1981). Who is the dreamer who dreams the dream and who is the dreamer who understands it? In: *Do I Dare Disturb the Universe?* London: Karnac.

Hakeem, A. (2007). Trans-sexuality. A case of the "Emperor's new clothes". In: D. Morgan & S. Ruszczynski (Eds.), *Lectures on Violence, Perversion and Delinquency*. London: Karnac.

Hill, D. (1994). The special place of the erotic transference in psychoanalysis. *Psycho-Analytic Inquiry*, *14*: 483–498.

Isaacs, S. (1952). The nature and function of phantasy. In: P. Heimann, S. Isaacs, M. Klein, & J. Riviere (Eds.), *Developments in Psychoanalysis*. London: Hogarth.

Israëls, H. (1989). *Schreber: Father and Son*. Madison, CT: International Universities Press.

Jacobs, W. J., & Nadel, L. (1985). Stress induced recovery of fears and phobias. *Psychological Review, 92*: 512–531.

Jaria, A. (1969). Contributo allo studio della pedofilia e delle sue implicanze psichiatrico-forensi. *Il lavoro neuropsichiatrico, 44*(3d).

Jiménez, J. P. (2006). After pluralism. Toward a new, integrated psychoanalytic paradigm. *International Journal of Psychoanalysis, 87*: 1487–1507.

Jones, E. (1953). *The Life and Work of Sigmund Freud*. New York: Basic Books, 1972.

Joseph, B. (1982). Addiction to near death. *International Journal of Psychoanalysis, 63*: 449–456.

Joseph, B. (1985). Transference. The total situation. *International Journal of Psychoanalysis, 66*: 447–454.

Kant, I. (2006[1798]). *Anthropology from a Pragmatic Point of View*, R. B. Louden (Trans.). Cambridge: Cambridge University Press.

Katan, M. (1954). The importance of the non-psychotic part of the personality in schizophrenia. *International Journal of Psychoanalysis, 35*: 119–128.

Kernberg, O. (1967). Borderline personality organization. *Journal of the American Psychoanalytic Association, 15*: 641–685.

Kernberg, O. (1975). *Borderline Conditions and Pathological Narcissism*. New York: Jason Aronson.

Kernberg, O. (1995). *Love Relations*. New Haven, CT: Yale University Press.

Kernberg, O. (2010). Transference focused psychotherapy (TFP). In: P. Williams (Ed.), *The Psychoanalytic Therapy of Severe Disturbance*. London: Karnac.

Kerr, J. (1993). *A Most Dangerous Method*. New York: Knopf.

Khan, M. (1963). *The Privacy of the Self*. London: Hogarth, 1974.

Khan, M. (1979). *Alienation in Perversion*. London: Hogarth.

Kim-Cohen, J., Caspi, A., Moffit, T. E., Harrington, H., Mine, B. J., & Poulton, R. (2003). Prior juvenile diagnoses in adults with mental disorder. Development follow-back of a prospective longitudinal cohort. *Archives of General Psychiatry, 60*: 709–717.

Klein, M. (1927a). Symposium on child analysis. *International Journal of Psychoanalysis, 8*: 377–380.

Klein, M. (1927b). Criminal tendencies in normal children. *British Journal of Medical Psychology, 7*: 177–192.

Klein, M. (1930). The importance of symbol-formation in the development of the ego. *International Journal of Psychoanalysis, 11*: 24–39.

Klein, M. (1932). *The Psycho-Analysis of Children*. London: Hogarth.

Klein, M. (1935). A contribution to the psychogenesis of manic-depressive states. *International Journal of Psychoanalysis, 16*: 145–174.

Klein, M. (1946). Notes on some schizoid mechanisms. *International Journal of Psychoanalysis, 27*: 99–110.

Klein, M. (1948). On the theory of anxiety and guilt. *International Journal of Psychoanalysis, 29*: 113–123.

Klein, M. (1950). *The Psychoanalysis of Children*. London: Hogarth.

Klein, M. (1955). On identification. In: M. Klein, P. Heimann, & R. Money-Kyrle (Eds.), *New Directions in Psycho-Analysis*. London: Tavistock.

Klein, M. (1963). Some reflections on "The Oresteia". In: *Our Adult World*. London: Heinemann.

Kohut, H. (1971). *The Analysis of the Self*. London: Hogarth Press.

Komisaruk, B., Beyer-Flores, C., & Whipple, B. (2006). *The Science of Orgasm*. Baltimore, MD: Johns Hopkins University Press.

LeDoux, J. (1996). *The Emotional Brain: The Mysterious Underpinnings of Emotional Life*. New York: Simon & Schuster.

Lemma, A. (2010). An order of pure decision. Growing up in a virtual world and the adolescent's experience of being a body. *Journal of the American Psychoanalytic Association, 4*: 691–714.

Levin, F. M. (2009). *Emotion and the Psychodynamic of the Cerebellum*. London: Karnac.

Limentani, A. (1979). The significance of transsexualism in relation to some basic psycho-analytic concepts. *International Review of Psychoanalysis, 6*: 139–153.

Lingiardi, V., & Madeddu, F. (2002). *I meccanismi di difesa. Teoria, valutazione, clinica*. Milan: Cortina.

Little, M. (1958). On delusional transference (transference psychosis). *International Journal of Psychoanalysis, 39*: 134–138.

Lombardi, R. (2003). Mental models and language registers in the psychoanalysis of psychosis. *International Journal of Psychoanalysis, 27*: 99–110.

Lombardi, R. (2005). On the psychoanalytic treatment of a psychotic patient. *Psychoanalytic Quarterly, 74*: 1069–1099.

London, N. J. (1973). An essay on psychoanalytic theory. Two theories of schizophrenia. *International Journal of Psychoanalysis, 54*: 169–193.

Lowenfels, W. (1962). Remembering Norman Douglas (for Nancy Cunard). *Literary Revue, 5*: 336–348.

Lubbe, T. (2008). A Kleinian theory of sexuality. *British Journal of Psychotherapy, 24*(3): 299–316.

Mann, T. (1995). *Death in Venice*, S. Appelbaum (Trans.). Mineola, NY: Dover Thrift Editions.

Masson, J. M. (Ed. & Trans.) (1985). *The Complete Letters of Sigmund Freud to Wilhelm Fliess, 1887–1904*. Cambridge, MA: The Belknap Press of Harvard University Press.

McDougall, J. (1995). *The Many Faces of Eros*. London: Free Association.

Meltzer, D. (1966). The relation of anal masturbation to projective identification. *International Journal of Psychoanalysis, 47*: 335–342.

Meltzer, D. (1973). *Sexual States of Mind*. Strathtay, Perthshire: Clunie Press.

Merciai, S. (2002). Psicoterapia online: un vestito su misura. In: Psychomedia (www.psychomedia.it/pm/pit/olpsy/merciai.htm) accessed on 28 December 2013.

Miller, A. (1983). *For Your Own Good: Hidden Cruelty in Child-Rearing and the Roots of Violence*, H. & H. Hannum (Trans.). London: Faber.

Modell, A. H. (1999). The dead mother syndrome and the reconstruction of trauma. In: G. Kohon (Ed.), *The Dead Mother* (pp. 76–86). London: Routledge.

Money-Kyrle, R. (1968). Cognitive development. *International Journal of Psychoanalysis, 49*: 691–698.

Money-Kyrle, R. (1971). The aim of psychoanalysis. *International Journal of Psychoanalysis, 52*: 103–106.

Nabokov, V. (1959). *Lolita*. London: Weidenfeld & Nicolson.

Niederland, W. G. (1951). Three notes on the Schreber case. *Psychoanalytic Quarterly, 20*: 579–591.

Oppenheimer, A. (1991). The wish for a sex change: a challenge to psychoanalysis? *International Journal of Psychoanalysis, 72*: 221–231.

O'Shaughnessy, E. (1981). A clinical study of a defensive organization. *International Journal of Psychoanalysis, 62*: 359–369.

Ovesey, L., & Person, E. S. (1973). Gender identity and sexual psychopathology in men. A psycho-dynamic analysis of homosexuality, transsexualism, and transvestism. *Journal of the American Academy of Psychoanalysis, 1*: 53–72.

Panel (1985). Sadomasochism in children. Fall meeting of the American Psychoanalytic Association, 2 December 1985.

Parens, H. (1997). The unique pathogenicity of sexual abuse. *Psychoanalytic Inquiry, 17*: 250–266.

Person, E. S. (1985). The erotic transference in women and in men: differences and coincidences. *Journal of the American Academy of Psychoanalysis, 13*: 159–180.

Pfäfflin, F. (2006). Research, research politics, and clinical experience with transsexual patients. In: P. Fonagy, M. Leuzinger-Bohleber, & R.

Krause (Eds.), *Identity, Gender, Sexuality. 150 Years after Freud.* London: Karnac.

Quinodoz, D. (1998). A fe/male transsexual patient in psychoanalysis. *International Journal of Psychoanalysis, 79*: 95–111.

Quinodoz, D. (2002). Termination of a fe/male transsexual patient's analysis. An example of general validity. *International Journal of Psychoanalysis, 83*: 783–798.

Racamier, P. C. (2000). Un espace pour délirer. *Revue Française de Psychanalise, 64*: 823–829.

Rappaport, E. A. (1959). The first dream of an erotized transference. *International Journal of Psychoanalysis, 40*: 240–245.

Raulet, G. (1991). The new utopia: communication technologies. *Telos, 87*: 39–58.

Resnik, S. (2001). *The Delusional Person: Bodily Feeling in Psychosis.* London: Karnac.

Rey, H. (1994). *Universals of Psychoanalysis in the Treatment of Psychotic and Borderline States,* J. Magagna (Ed.). London: Free Association.

Rizzolatti, G., Fogassi, L., & Gallese, V. (2001). Neurophysiological mechanisms underlying the understanding and imitation of action. *Neuroscience, 2*: 661–670.

Rosenfeld, H. (1964). On the psychopathology of narcissism. A clinical approach. *International Journal of Psychoanalysis, 45*: 332–337.

Rosenfeld, H. (1971). A clinical approach to the psychoanalytic theory of life and death instincts. An investigation into aggressive aspects of narcissism. *International Journal of Psychoanalysis, 52*: 169–177.

Rosenfeld, H. (1978). Notes on the psychopathology and psychoanalytic treatment of some borderline patients. *International Journal of Psychoanalysis, 58*: 215–223.

Rosenfeld, H. (1979). Transference psychosis. In: J. LeBoit & A. Capponi (Eds.), *Advances in Psychotherapy of the Borderline Patient.* New York: Jason Aronson.

Rosenfeld, H. (1987). *Impasse and Interpretation.* London: Tavistock.

Rosenfeld, H. (2001). *Herbert Rosenfeld at Work,* F. De Masi (Ed.). London: Karnac.

Sacher-Masoch, L. von (1947). *Venus in Furs.* New York: Sylvan Press.

Sade, D. A. F. de (1991[1784]). The one hundred and twenty days of Sodom. In: A. Wainhau & R. Seaver (Comp. & Trans.), *The One Hundred and Twenty Days of Sodom and Other Writings.* London: Arrow.

Sandler, J., & Sandler, A. M. (1987). The past unconscious, the present unconscious and the vicissitudes of guilt. *International Journal of Psychoanalysis, 68*: 331–341.

Schafer, R. (1977). The interpretation of transference and the conditions for loving. *Journal of the American Psychoanalytic Association, 25*: 335–362.

Schmitt, C. (2007[1963]). *Theory of the Partisan: Intermediate Commentary on the Concept of the Political by Carl Schmitt*, G. L. Ulmen (Trans.). New York: Telos Press.

Schore, A. N. (2003). *Affect Regulation and the Repair of the Self*. New York: Norton.

Schreber, D. P. (1955). *Memoirs of My Nervous Illness*, I. Macalpine & R. Hunter (Eds. & Trans.). London: Dawson.

Scoville, W. B., & Milner, B. (1957). Loss of the recent memory after bilateral hippocampal lesions. *Journal of Neurology, Neurosurgery and Psychiatry, 20*: 11–21.

Searles, H. F. (1963). Transference psychosis in the psychotherapy of schizophrenia. *International Journal of Psychoanalysis, 44*: 249–281.

Segal, H. (1956). Depression in the schizophrenic. *International Journal of Psychoanalysis, 37*: 339–343.

Segal, H. (1991). *Dream, Phantasy and Art*. London: Routledge.

Socarides, C. W. (1959). Meaning and content of a paedophilic perversion. *Journal of the American Psychoanalytic Association, 7*: 84–94.

Solms, M. (2006). An interview. Mark D. Smaller. *American Psychoanalyst, 40*: 1.

Sparti, D. (2000). *Wittgenstein politico*. Milan: Feltrinelli.

Spensley, S. (2006). Commentary to the paper "Developmental research on childhood gender identity disorder" of Susan Coates. In: P. Fonagy, M. Leuzinger-Bohleber, & R. Krause (Eds.), *Identity, Gender, Sexuality. 150 Years after Freud*. London: Karnac.

Spillius, E. B. (1983). Some developments from the work of Melanie Klein. *International Journal of Psychoanalysis, 64*: 321–332.

Stein, R. (1995). Analysis of a case of transsexualism. *Psychoanalytic Dialogues, 5*: 257–289.

Stein, R. (1998). The poignant, the excessive and the enigmatic in sexuality. *International Journal of Psychoanalysis, 79*: 253–268.

Steiner, J. (1982). Relationships between parts of the self. *International Journal of Psychoanalysis, 63*: 241–251.

Steiner, J. (1993). *Psychic Retreats. Pathological Organizations in Psychotic, Neurotic and Borderline Patients*. London: Routledge.

Stern, D. (1985). *The Motherhood Constellation. A Unified View of Parent–Infant Psychotherapy*. London: Karnac.

Stoller, R. (1964). The hermaphroditic identity of hermaphrodites. *Journal of Nervous and Mental Disease, 139*(5): 453–457.

Stoller, R. (1968). Male child transsexualism. *Journal of the American Academy of Psycho-analysis, 7:* 193–201.

Stoller, R. (1975). *Perversion. The Erotic Form of Hatred.* New York: Pantheon Books.

Stolorow, R. D., & Atwood, G. E. (1992). *Context of Being. The Intersubjective Foundations of the Psychic Life.* Hillsdale, NJ: Analytic Press.

Sulloway, F. (1979). *Freud, Biologist of the Mind: Beyond the Psychoanalytic Legend.* New York: Basic Books.

Sylvester, D. (1998). *Interviews with Francis Bacon: The Brutality of Fact.* London: Thames and Hudson.

The Mahabharata of Krishna-Dwaipayana Vyasa, K. M. Ganguli (Trans.). Accessed at the Internet Sacred Text Archive, www.sacred-texts.com/hin/maha/index.htm, on 28 December 2013.

Thomä, H., & Kächele, H. (1985). *Leherbuch der psychoanalytischen Therapie.* 1. Berlin-Heidelberg: Springer (*Psychoanalytic Practice, 1.* Berlin-Heidelberg: Springer; *Psychoanalytic Practice, 2.* Berlin-Heidelberg: Springer, 1988).

Tronick, E. (1989). Emotions and emotional communication in infants. *American Psychologist, 44:* 112–119.

Tsolas, V. (2007). Transference love and the treatment of a pre-surgical male transvestite. IPA Congress, Berlin.

Vallario, L. (2008). *Naufraghi nella rete.* Milan: Franco Angeli.

Van der Kolk, B. A. (1994). The body keeps the score. Memory and evolving psychobiology of post-traumatic stress. *Harvard Review of Psychiatry, Mosby-Year Book, 1:* 263–265.

Van der Kolk, B. A., McFarlane, A., & Weisaeth, L. (1996). *Traumatic Stress: The Effects of Overwhelming Experience on Mind, Body, and Society.* New York: Guilford Press.

Wallerstein, R. S. (1967). Reconstruction and mastery in the transference psychosis. *International Journal of Psychoanalysis, 15:* 551–583.

Weinshel, E. M. (1966). Severe regressive states during analysis. *International Journal of Psychoanalysis, 16:* 538–568.

Williams, A. H. (1998). *Cruelty, Violence and Murder: Understanding the Criminal Mind.* London: Jason Aronson.

Williams, P. (2004). Incorporation of an invasive object. *International Journal of Psychoanalysis, 85:* 1333–1348.

Williams, P. (2010). *The Fifth Principle.* London: Karnac.

Winnicott, D. W. (1949). Hate in the counter-transference. *International Journal of Psychoanalysis, 30:* 69–74.

Winnicott, D. W. (1971). *Playing and Reality.* London: Tavistock.

Winnicott, D. W. (1975). *Through Paediatrics to Psycho-Analysis: Collected Papers*. New York: Basic Books.

Winnicott, D. W. (1989). *Psycho-Analytic Explorations*. London: Karnac.

Young, K. S. (1998). Internet addiction. The emergence of a new clinical disorder. *CyberPsychology and Behavior, 1*: 237–244.

Yovell, Y. (2000). From hysteria to posttraumatic stress disorder. Psychoanalysis and the neurobiology of traumatic memories. *Neuro-Psychoanalysis, 2*: 171–181.

Zanzotto, A. (2007). *Eterna riabilitazione da un trauma di cui si ignora la natura*, L. Barile & G. Bompiani (Eds.). Rome: Edizione Nottetempo.

INDEX